D0829051

The Patient's Guide to Weight Loss Surgery

The Patient's Guide to Weight Loss Surgery

Everything You Need to Know about Gastric Bypass and Bariatric Surgery

April Hochstrasser, PhD
with a Foreword by S. Ross Fox, MD

A Healthy Living Book
Hatherleigh Press
5–22 46th Avenue, Suite 200
Long Island City, NY 11101
www.healthylivingbooks.com

Library of Congress Cataloging-in-Publication Data

Hochstrasser, April.
  The patient's guide to weight loss surgery : everything you need to know about gastric bypass and bariatric surgery / April Hochstrasser, with a foreword by S. Ross Fox.
     p. cm.
  "A Healthy Living Book."
  Includes index.
  ISBN 1-57826-165-1
  1. Obesity--Surgery--Popular works. 2. Gastric bypass--Popular works. 3. Weight loss--Popular works. I. Title.
  RD540.H63 2004
  617.4'3--dc22
                        2004008131

Healthy Living Books titles are available for bulk purchase, special promotions, and premiums. For information about reselling and special purchase opportunities, please call 1-800-528-2550 and ask for the Special Sales Manager.

Cover and interior design by Deborah Miller.
Illustrations by April Hochstrasser

10 9 8 7 6 5 4 3
Printed in Canada

Contents

Chapter 1. Types of Weight Loss Surgery 1

Overview • Vertical Banded Gastroplasty • Gastric Bypass • Fobi-Pouch Operation • Mini/Loop Gastric Bypass • Adjustable Gastric Band • Bileopancreatic Diversion • Jejuno-Ileal Bypass • Implantable Gastric Stimulation System • Gastric Balloon • Mortality Rates • How Big Is the Mature Pouch? • Summary

Chapter 2. What Changing Your Body Image May Mean 31

Body Types • Metropolitan Insurance Company Weight Tables • Paradigm Shift about Food • Somatoform Personality Types • Surgical Remedies and their Consequences • Prejudice Against Fat People • Emotional Considerations • Controlling Thoughts and Feelings • Positive Aspects of Weight Loss Surgery

Chapter 3. Negative Aspects of the Surgery 47

Risks of Malnutrition • Risks of Weight Loss Surgery

List of Illustrations

List of Abbreviations

Abbreviations
AGB   Adjustable Gastric Band
BPD   Bileopancreatic Diversion
BMI   Body Mass Index
CCK   Cholecystokinin
DS   Duodenal Switch
FPO   Fobi-Pouch Operation
GBP   Gastric Bypass
IGS   Implantable Gastric Stimulation System
ISAA   International Size Acceptance Association
NIH   National Institutes Of Health
RNY   Roux-en-Y Gastric Bypass
SRVG   Silastic Ring Vertical Gastroplasty
VBG   Vertical Banded Gastroplasty
WLS   Weight Loss Surgery

Foreword

Obesity: America's Modern-Day Plague

In medieval times, millions of people died from bubonic plague. It was a disease associated with squalor. Today the plague killing Americans is obesity, and it is a disease of affluence. According to the National Institutes of Health (NIH), overweight is the leading cause of preventable death in this country. A million Americans die of it every three and a half years. That is 300,000 each year. This is the equivalent of two fully loaded 747s crashing into the side of a mountain every day. Sixty-one percent of American adults are overweight, and obesity has become the country's most serious leading public health problem.

A great majority of Americans who are heavy are that way primarily because of their genetics. It is true that they must consume the calories to put on the weight, but their biology asks them to do that. When their excess weight reaches around 100 pounds, it is virtually impossible for them to get the weight off and keep it off without drastic interventions.

The NIH has looked at various therapies for the treatment of morbid obesity (100 pounds or more overweight) on several occasions in the past 30 years, and has found that diet, exercise, behavior modification, and other treatments are virtually never successful. The NIH has stated that the most effective therapy for long-term significant weight loss in morbidly obese patients is surgery. This sentiment has been echoed by Dr. C. Everett Koop, the American Academy of Science, and other prestigious scientific groups.

Along with morbid obesity comes a myriad of serious, often life-threatening medical problems—we call them comorbidities—all of which are either entirely relieved or markedly improved by undergoing obesity surgery. But of all the benefits of weight loss surgery, the most significant is the heightened quality of life that patients experience. As their disabilities disappear, along with their significant medical problems, all aspects of life improve dramatically!

While bariatric (obesity) surgery is radical therapy, and there are some risks associated with it (very minimal), the results in the great majority of patients are very impressive. But bariatric surgery is only a tool that enables a patient to control her or his morbid obesity, and the tool must be used properly.

Regular follow-up of the patients is mandatory to achieve the best results. Patients who avail themselves of the opportunity for careful follow-up rarely have significant long-term complications, and their statement commonly is, "I would do it again in a heartbeat."

In a patient's search for a surgeon to perform an obesity operation, I always recommend that they find someone who has done hundreds of the operations and who has an excellent long-term follow-up program including support groups, dietary counseling, and psychological help if needed. When such a surgeon is found, the results are usually very impressive. Many of the surgeon's patients will say, "You have given my life back to me."

If you are heavy, this book is about making an informed decision to 'get your life back.'

S. Ross Fox, MD

former President, American Society for Bariatric Surgery

Author's Note

This book is about weight loss surgery. It neither advocates nor discourages surgery, but seeks to give the reader a realistic picture of what might be expected from these procedures.

The book is divided into three sections. The first section is an overview of the different types of surgery available; the costs, the techniques, the possible reasons for having the surgery, as well as potential side effects. The second part of the book discusses healthy attitudes toward weight and weight loss, and pragmatic solutions for weight control. The third part of the book is devoted to telling the stories of people who have had this surgery. Accounts of both successful and traumatic outcomes are included so that the reader will have an idea of the range of experiences in weight loss surgery. The goal of the book is to help the reader make the best decision regarding the appropriateness of weight loss surgery for his or her individual circumstances and personality.

Acknowledgments

I would like to acknowledge the following people who have helped immeasurably with this book: Michael Bateman, MD, who encouraged me in this field; Steve Hawks, PhD, who gave essential organizational suggestions and graciously previewed the book when it was still rough; Anthony Brand, mentor with Fairfax, University, UK; Mikaela Griggs and Debbie Gessel for their editing skills; Dr. Susan Morris and Karen Anderson for their support; Dr. S. Ross Fox for help with medical refinements and the Foreword; and my husband, Gary Hochstrasser, for his support of me in whatever I want to do in life.

1

Types of Weight-Loss Surgery

Currently, four major types of stomach surgery exist: the Vertical Banded Gastroplasty (VBG), the Gastric Bypass (GBP), also called the Roux-en-Y Gastric Bypass (RNY), the Adjustable Gastric Band (AGB), and the Bileopancreatic Diversion (BPD). In addition, some experimental procedures are now being developed. These surgeries are performed worldwide in university centers and private hospitals and have been remarkably successful in providing significant weight loss. In 2002 there were 94,000 procedures in the United States and approximately 140,000 in 2003. In general, these procedures are most appropriate for severely obese patients between 15 and 70 years of age, who have attempted medical management of their obesity but have been unsuccessful in achieving permanent weight loss.[1]

Surgical treatment does not involve removal of adipose (fat) tissue by suction or excision. Instead, the size of the gastric reservoir (stomach) is reduced with or without re-routing the intestines. Eating behavior thus improves dramatically because the person can no longer comfortably hold as much food. This reduces caloric intake and ensures that the patient practices behavior modification, eats small amounts slowly, and chews each mouthful well.[2]

To be a candidate for insurance coverage, it is often necessary that the patient have other medical problems such as arthritis, back or disc disease, diabetes, elevated serum cholesterol, fatigue, hypertension, hiatal hernia, gallbladder disease, shortness of breath, or significant disability. Generally, the more medical problems a person has, the more likely it is their medical insurance will provide part or full coverage for the surgery. Some insurance policies that will not cover other diet and weight control programs may cover this surgery if medical need (comorbidity) can be demonstrated.

In general, patients must be at least 100 pounds overweight or have a BMI greater than 40 (see Chapter 10). Doctors usually set the limit at 100 pounds, but some insurance companies require double the expected weight. Thus, a person who should weigh 150 pounds would be eligible for this surgery at 250 pounds. However, their insurance policy might require that the person weigh 300 pounds for the surgery to be covered; insurance companies set the guidelines arbitrarily. This surgery is considered a last resort as treatment for obesity and should be done only after other programs have been seriously tried without success. The heaviest person Dr. Ross Fox, a well-known bariatric doctor, has operated on weighed 750 pounds. Denied a seat on an airplane, a bus and also a train because of his weight, this person had to be driven across the country in an automobile to receive the surgery. Other bariatric doctors have reported operating on bed-ridden patients weighing as much as 800 pounds or more.

The youngest person on whom the surgery has been performed was reported to be pre-adolescent. That child, already

200 pounds overweight, had made numerous attempts at losing weight, had attended diet camps and was, prior to the surgery, not going to school, but sitting at home and playing video games. Lifestyle options for that child changed dramatically following surgery.

Prejudice against a severely obese teenager or child is enormous. Morbidly obese children may withdraw from society and/or their own feelings in an attempt to protect themselves, and they may even attempt suicide.

Vertical Banded Gastroplasty (VBG)

This procedure is a gastric restrictive operation that involves the creation of a small stomach within the normal stomach, which would ordinarily hold 4 to 6 cups of food. In VBG, a line of staples is placed high on the right side of the stomach, forming a pouch. Better results seem to come from actually severing a portion of the stomach to prevent staple line failure (when the staples do not hold the pouch together), but this complicates a relatively simple operation. The outlet to the new stomach is carefully measured and its size is precisely controlled. The newly created "small stomach" ranges from 10 cc to 30 cc in size. (30 cc is approximately the same size as a shot glass.) An unaltered stomach holds 4 to 6 cups of food. The outlet from this small pouch is also smaller than the outlet from the normal stomach, (one-fourth to one-half inch), to allow the contents of the smaller stomach to drain more slowly into the larger stomach below it.

A Marlex mesh band or Silastic ring (non-stretchable reinforcers) is placed around the outlet of the pouch formed by the gastric partition. The importance of the band or ring is to keep the outlet from stretching. The staple line is vertically oriented,

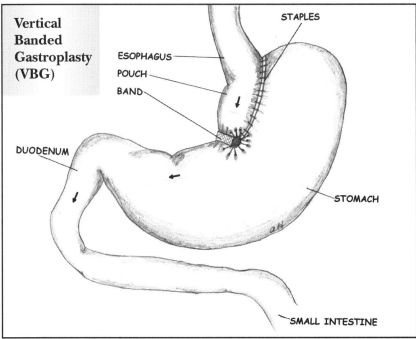

Vertical Banded Gastroplasty (VBG)

STAPLES

ESOPHAGUS

POUCH

BAND

DUODENUM

STOMACH

SMALL INTESTINE

Illustration 1-1

hence the name Vertical Banded Gastroplasty, also called the Lap-Band.

There has been a decrease in the use of VBG since 1995, one of the reasons being that it is generally an open operation and not done laparoscopically. However, the incidence of common complications associated with other surgical choices is greatly diminished with VGB. Patients who undergo VGB have a much lower risk of developing iron deficiency, anemia, osteoporosis, osteomalacia, hyperparathyroidism, stomach ulcer, duodenal ulcer, obstruction of the GI tract and the Dumping Syndrome (see page 11). Most patients are able to drink milk and absorb the calcium and vitamin D to help avoid bone disease as they age.[3]

When food in the small pouch empties into the larger stomach, gastric juices mix with the food and digestion continues, with normal passage into the small intestine. People eat less because they feel full after consuming a very small quantity of food.

Many patients feel pressure or tightness in their upper chest when they overeat, even by only one or two tablespoons of food. This feeling of fullness is uncomfortable for many post-operative patients, and the sensation leads some to try and thwart the effectiveness of the band. Eating tiny bites and chewing thoroughly is a hard habit to acquire when a person is accustomed to eating for volume. New struggles arise as these patients can no longer eat the quantities they are used to. It can be frustrating to leave most of the food on the plate virtually untouched when one is still hungry.

Drinking a lot of water with each bite and liquefying the food before swallowing can sabotage the band. For this reason, doctors recommend drinking no liquid with meals and chewing more than usual to create a softer bolus (food ball). Some patients soon learn to eat wet foods, such as salads with oily dressing or creamy macaroni and cheese, because these pass easily through the band, thus keeping weight loss to a minimum.

Others sabotage this procedure by continuing to eat high-calorie foods that liquefy quickly, such as ice cream and puddings. These foods don't stay in the small pouch that has been created, so the patient can keep on eating. It is the feeling of fullness, and the subsequent slower emptying of the small stomach, that lead to weight loss when the patient is forced to eat small meals. Overeating can result in vomiting, gagging and a very uncomfortable feeling that causes some to try and throw up the food that feels like an "egg stuck in the throat." Throwing up the three to four tablespoons of food that have been eaten is easy if it is still in the small stomach pouch, but impossible if it has passed to the larger stomach. However, if an illness forces a person to throw up, the body finds a way to make it happen, even from the larger stomach portion beyond the restriction. There may be an increased risk of gastric reflux if the patient continues to overeat. Therefore a clear understanding of, and commitment to, the lifestyle changes that will be required following this surgery must be accepted by the patient.

Vertical banded gastroplasty can be reversed by unfastening the staples used to section off the small stomach. This common procedure returns the stomach to its regular size, resulting in the regaining of weight. In creating the small gastric pouch, fluids must still pass through easily or the patient will become dehydrated. Unfortunately, a number of fluids available to us in our society are high-calorie and include foods such as ice cream, milk, soda, and other sweetened beverages. If VBG patients do not avoid high-calorie liquids, they will not lose as much weight as they would if these foods were avoided. Successful VBG patients have learned to stay away from these foods. There is no other disruption of the intestinal tract with VGB, aside from the creation of the small pouch and partitioning with the band.

A study of the long-term effects of the gastric band reports a dissatisfaction level approaching 58 percent because of failure to lose the expected amount of weight.[4] Vertical banded gastroplasty will benefit a selected number of individuals, but the super morbidly obese may not be able to lose enough weight from a restrictive surgical procedure.

DEFINITIONS

Morbidly obese: Patients whose body weight exceeds the healthy limit by 100 pounds with a BMI between 40 and 50.

Super morbidly obese: Those whose body weight exceeds the healthy limit by more than 200 pounds with a BMI over 50.

Those with a history of bulimia will be unable to force themselves to vomit after the procedure—possibly resulting in an increase of other compulsive behaviors. They can still vomit the contents of the small pouch, but that will only be a few tablespoons of food. Those who already like to eat smaller snacks throughout the day will not experience as much success because this procedure invites consumption of many tiny meals. Those who control their moods with comfort foods may feel anxious when those foods are denied them. Comfort foods can be any food associated with pleasant memories; they are, however, most often soft, high-density, high-fat and sweet, like peanut butter and jelly, or ice cream. The comfort of a nursing baby may subconsciously be sought from the taste and texture of comfort foods.

After VBG surgery, the patient needs to consume two to five high-protein liquid meals a day for the first weeks; solid foods are then gradually added. The size of a typical solid food meal is about the size of a one ounce shot glass, but the liquid diet can be one or two cups of liquid. Hunger may be experienced because the small stomach doesn't stay full very long. Five years after this surgery is performed, the average patient has lost less than 50 percent of his or her total weight loss goal. This is generally the lowest average among the four procedures.

The hospital stay for VBG is 1 to 2 days, and convalescence at home is 1 to 3 weeks. Convalescence depends on the original health of the patient and any complications that may arise during or after the procedure.[5]

Between one-third and one-half of the patients who undergo VBG come back later for a more drastic surgical intervention. Eventually, they may opt for a gastric bypass, so that fewer calories are absorbed and more weight can be lost.

It is possible to unfasten the staples used in the procedure if the patient wants to reverse the surgery, and often the staples unfasten themselves over time. Once the staples are removed, the stomach returns to its original size. In most cases, the patient then regains the weight that was lost.

New staplers, such as the SurgAssist Stapler, have been available only since 2002. These new staplers make staple lines 2 1/2 times stronger than the old devices, which doctors have used for 20 years. Patients should ask their doctor if they use the newest technology available, because staple failure and subsequent leakage is one of the most common complications of WLS.

Variations of Vertical Banded Gastroplasty

Vertical banded gastroplasty procedures can be performed laparoscopically, using trocars and laparoscopes as an alternative to invasive surgery. This involves placing cameras and instruments into the body through several small one-inch slits, rather than a long open incision. Another variation involves cutting the stomach and removing a small V shape, then stapling it, but allowing the two sections to heal with scar tissue. This new V-shaped scar line is stronger than the staples, and eliminates the possibility of the staples coming out later. (See Illustration 1-1 on page 4.)

Gastric Bypass (GBP)

The Gastric Bypass was developed by Dr. Edward Mason in the 1960s and was named because the food that is eaten bypasses the major portion of the stomach and a generous length of the small intestine. Food is not absorbed until it mixes with gastric juices

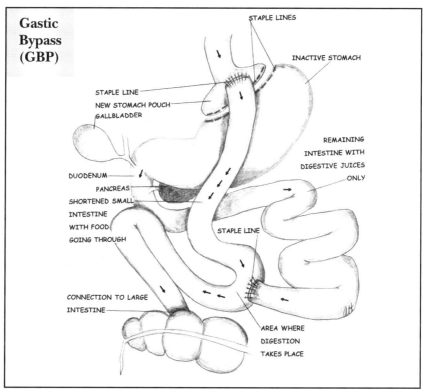

Illustration 1-2

farther down in an artificially created juncture in the intestines. Some of the food that is eaten is not digested, but is passed through the system. This food does not supply nutrients and cause accumulation of fat.

The Gastric Bypass, also called Roux Gastric Bypass or the Roux-en-Y Gastric Bypass, is a procedure in which a small gastric pouch is made in the same part of the upper stomach as in VBG. However, the stomach is then severed at that point and forms scar tissue once healed. The larger portion of the stomach is sealed off and the outlet to the small intestine remains, even though there is now no top access to this part of the stomach. This leaves a small, blind pouch into which food arrives from the esophagus. The pouch is blind because it has no outlet. The "plumbing," or the exit from this part of the stomach is then changed.) The first part of the small intestine, the duodenum, is about 12 inches long; the jejunum is 60 to 90 inches long, and the last part of the intestine, the ileum, is 110 to 120 inches long. This totals almost 20 feet of small intestine. A piece of small intestine is cut and brought up to attach to the pouch, so that food can exit from the pouch into the segment of the small intestine that is now connected. There is an increase in the risk of leakage for the first few days after surgery until the scar tissue forms.

With the most radical distal bypass, the intestine is cut so all that remains is 40 to 60 inches of the bottom portion of the small intestine (ileum), where food is absorbed. The new top portion of intestine conducts food from the pouch to the new junction, but does not absorb food. Vitamins and minerals can be absorbed in the upper length of intestine but, because of the lack of gastric juices, food cannot. The larger stomach is now used to conduct gastric juices to the Y–shaped junction. Until the gastric juices are introduced at the artificial juncture, food is not absorbed into the bloodstream. The reattached portion of the small intestine from the pouch joins the original small intestine forming a Y shape. (See Illustration 1–2 on page 9.) Then the digestive juices and bile from the stomach, gallbladder, liver, and pancreas mix with the food at this artificial point and digestion occurs.

There is no change in the connection from small intestine to large intestine. Almost no absorption of food occurs in the large intestine (colon) but it primarily helps regulate hydration levels in the body.

This last segment of the small intestine provides the only opportunity the body has to digest food. Much of the food goes into the colon (large intestine) undigested. As a result of the small stomach pouch—which restricts the amount of food that can be consumed—and the reduced intestinal tract—which limits the amount of nutrient absorption—the patient loses weight. This may result in malnutrition unless a strict adherence to a lifetime of protein drinks and supplements is maintained.[6] Although normally preventable and treatable, GBP can result in iron, calcium, and vitamin B-12 deficiencies as well as other vitamin and mineral deficiencies.

A major side effect of a gastric bypass operation is that patients tolerate sweets poorly. A GBP patient who eats anything with a significant amount of sugar in it will feel lightheaded and experience palpitations (heart flutters) as well as cold sweats. Although these symptoms only last for a few minutes, they are very unpleasant and have been named the Dumping Syndrome. Dumping is a physiological reaction to a high sugar load. When a lot of sugar quickly enters the small intestine, the body senses the sugar level rising and "dumps" insulin to handle the load. This dramatically lowers blood sugar and can result in nausea, vomiting, cramping, flushing and a sense of fear and uneasiness as well as the above-mentioned symptoms. This range of negative reactions is sufficient to condition most people against eating sweets. This phenomenon usually lasts for one to three years after surgery, until the body adjusts to the change. However, for some people the syndrome is permanent, and they are never able to consume sugar in any form again without consequences. For this reason, the GBP operation is usually more successful than the VBG if the patient is a sweet-eater.

Other nutritional complications that may occur are low serum protein levels and anemia. There is also a possibility of gastric ulcers forming at the juncture of the pouch and the small intestine. The other less pleasant side effects of GBP can include diarrhea, constipation or malodorous gas. There can also be leaking junctures where cuts were made and tissue re-attached.

Additional complications related to these surgeries can include adhesions, when tissues stick together; bowel obstruction, when bowels don't function properly because of a blockage; and embolisms, which are blood clots and vessel obstructions. Potential disasters with anesthesia and infections can be complications as well. The choice between operations relates somewhat to a person's feeling about sugar and their ability to avoid it. Following GBP, patients usually stay in the hospital 1 to 3 days, followed by convalescence at home for 1 to 3 weeks, depending on the patient's overall health and the incidence of side effects. Some patients cannot return to normal activities for as long as six weeks, while others are back to work in a week. Following most obesity surgeries, dietary supplements, vitamins, minerals and protein drinks are necessary each day for the rest of the person's life. Regular laboratory studies and lifetime follow-up are also mandatory.

Of the patients who die after gastric bypass, half die due to technical complications, whereas the other half die of complications of their obesity. Only 20 percent of patients were suspected to have pulmonary emboli; yet at autopsy, 80 percent of bariatric patients had pulmonary emboli. In morbidly obese patients undergoing gastric bypass, there is an unexpectedly high rate of clinically silent pulmonary emboli contributing to morbidity and mortality.[7]

Variations of Gastric Bypass

There are three variations of this procedure that have some effect on outcome and side effects.

Distal Gastric Bypass. In this procedure the small intestine is attached as in GBP, and only the least amount of intestine that can safely be left for adequate absorption of food and nutrients remains. Patients who opt to have the least amount of about 40 inches must be willing to take their supplements and protein shakes religiously or experience malnutrition. A length of 60 inches is usually thought to be safer for the majority of people. After five years, the average patient will have maintained a 70 to 80 percent weight loss. However, this procedure carries the greatest risk for complications such as malnutrition, dehydration and gas. With the distal bypass, frequent uncontrollable gas is more serious than with the medial or proximal procedures. If gas is serious, the patient can be given an antibiotic to stave off the bacteria that causes gas in the colon.

Medial Gastric Bypass. In this procedure, the stomach contents mix with the gastric juices at the middle of the small intestine. There is a longer chamber of small intestine for the food to pass through and be absorbed. After five years, the patient will have maintained 50 to 60 percent of the total amount of weight they wanted to lose.

Proximal Gastric Bypass. In this variation of GBP, the small intestine segments are joined closer to the stomach, and only a small section of the small intestine is not used for digestion. After five years, the patients who undergo this procedure have maintained a 50 percent or less weight loss from their original goal weight, but this procedure is safer in terms of future problems with malnutrition. Because a major portion of the small intestine remains intact, the patient is less likely to suffer severe forms of nutrient deficiency and malnutrition than with the more radical distal bypass. Problems with diarrhea and gas are also minimized with the proximal bypass. However, this procedure is more likely to result in eventual weight regain as the body adjusts to its new bowel configuration.

In all the GBP operations, the patient has a window of time (12 to 24 months) in which to lose weight before the body becomes accustomed to the new caloric amount and adjusts itself accordingly. There is usually very little weight lost after 24 months. The person may struggle to maintain the lost weight just as they did before the surgery.

Fobi-Pouch Operation

The Fobi-Pouch Operation (FPO) is a variation of the traditional GBP. It was originally performed on patients who did not lose enough weight from the VBG but who already had a Marlex band or Silastic ring around the upper portion of the stomach. Dr. Mathias Fobi, who created this procedure, left these bands and rings in place and converted the operation into a gastric bypass. He found that stretching of the outlet was minimized when contained by the bands or rings. The Fobi-Pouch also refers to placing a synthetic ring around the tiny outlet when a previous surgery has not been done. This extends the time required to empty the pouch. The decision to place a ring around the outlet is a deeply divisive issue in bariatric surgery, but no solid data exist to support or refute this procedure.

Mini Gastric Bypass or Loop Gastric Bypass

This procedure is similar to the gastric bypass, with one major difference—the intestine is not severed and reconnected.

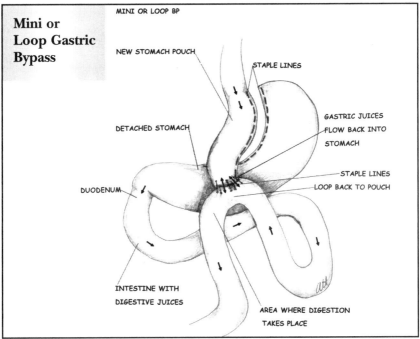

Illustration 1-3

Instead, after leaving the lower stomach section the intestine is looped back up and connected to the small upper pouch by making a new opening into it. (See Illustration 1-3, above). The gastric juices that normally mix with the stomach content after leaving the stomach are re-routed back into the stomach, causing it to be bathed in bile and pancreatic juices. This results in an increase in biliary reflux gastritis in more than 50 percent of patients. This mixing normally occurs in the intestine farther away from the delicate stomach lining. The opportunity for intestinal juices to go back into the stomach can result in severe heartburn, ulcers and inflammation of the esophagus.[8] This procedure is not performed by most bariatric doctors because of proven long-term side effects that cannot be adequately overcome. However, because of the relative ease of the procedure, in some cases taking less than 30 minutes, there are clinics that specialize in it. It is becoming more popular despite the side effects.

Adjustable Gastric Band (AGB)

The Adjustable Gastric Band is the newest approved technology in obesity surgery. It was approved for use in the USA in June of 2001. The original investigative study, conducted in the early 1990s, was sponsored by the U.S. Food and Drug Administration (FDA) and several American clinics. Patients who have had this surgery as a part of that study, or who have traveled outside the United States to have the surgery, have exhibited impressive results. Five years after the surgery, the average patient who had adjusted to eating 3 to 9 ounces of food at a time had lost 50 to 70 percent of the weight he or she originally wanted to lose.

In Adjustable Gastric Band surgery, an inflatable silicone band is placed laparoscopically (without a major incision) around the upper stomach. With laparoscopic surgery, several inch-long slits are made through the patient's abdominal wall instead of a major incision several inches long. The surgery is performed through these slits with the aid of small cameras that are also inserted in the slits, allowing the surgeon to view the surgery on a TV screen. It is imperative that an experienced surgeon perform this operation because vision is reduced when the stomach is not exposed. The surgeon also has no tactile sense when using remotely controlled instruments to guide him or her.

Regardless of the method of surgery, the procedure involves a silicone band. When in place, the band squeezes around the upper part of the stomach, creating a small pouch. The smaller pouch at the top is connected to the larger stomach through a small, banded tunnel. The advantage of the band is that if a person does not lose enough weight, the band can easily be adjusted in the physician's office by adding sterile water to inflate and tighten it. This facilitates greater weight loss, as less food is allowed to empty out of the small pouch, and at a slower rate.

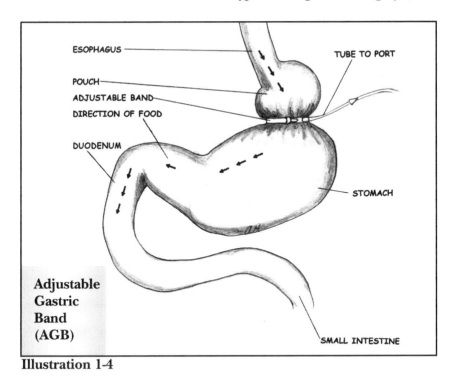

ESOPHAGUS

TUBE TO PORT

POUCH

ADJUSTABLE BAND

DIRECTION OF FOOD

DUODENUM

STOMACH

**Adjustable
Gastric
Band
(AGB)**

SMALL INTESTINE

Illustration 1-4

In the office procedure, sterile water or a saline solution, (called a "fill," or an "adjustment") is inserted into or taken out of the adjustable band. The band connects by tubing to a port, which can be felt just under the skin in the chest or side. This is a permanent site where the surgeon can add or remove water from the band that constricts the stomach. This internal tubing can be adjusted by tightening or loosening without going back into the abdomen surgically. If a person is losing weight too quickly or losing too much, the band can be loosened by taking out some of the water, and then the food will pass more easily into the full stomach area.

The bariatric surgeon does the adjustment by administering a local anesthetic, and then inserting a needle through the skin and into the "port" that accesses the band. The needle can suck water out to loosen the tightness of the band, or can insert a few ccs of water to tighten it. (See Illustration 1–4 on page 17.)

When the AGB is performed laparoscopically, patients can be in the hospital 24 hours or less. In the past, persons who wanted this particular surgery were sent to competent centers around the world; they then received specialized follow-up care in United States universities or clinic centers that normally perform other gastric procedures. Now, the whole procedure and follow-up can be done in the United States, although it is sometimes less expensive to have the procedure in another country. Insurance may not pay for this procedure because some insurance carriers still consider it to be experimental.

The AGB is not a magic bullet, and the patient must relearn his or her eating habits to lose weight. Patients report feeling frustrated at being put on a diet after this procedure. They must learn to be content with tiny portions even though they may still want more. The hunger peptide, ghrelin, is not reduced because the stomach remains intact; therefore hunger signals may be as strong as they were before surgery. Drinking high-calorie liquids or eating excessive amounts of soup, yogurt or pudding will result in a minimal weight loss and not cause a feeling of fullness. This procedure does not cause malabsorption, and whatever the patient eats is converted to energy and/or fat. The patient can expect to lose 5 to 10 pounds a month with the AGB after the first couple of months of rapid weight loss. They may be advised to give up all milk and sugar and may have difficulty eating red meat, pasta, white bread and sticky rice because these get "stuck" and cause an uncomfortable feeling of blockage. Patients are also advised to begin an exercise program if possible. AGB is a tool that can help in losing weight, though the nutritional guidelines given by the doctor must be strictly adhered to—and many feel these are another diet. A long-term satisfaction study of the adjustable gastric band done in Belgium reported about a 20 percent failure of the patients to lose any weight.[9]

If a patient's medical insurance doesn't cover obesity surgery, the AGB may be an excellent option for relief of serious obesity when performed outside the United States, and would then cost about half as much. Currently, AGB in Mexico costs $7,000 to $10,000, (not including the cost of the necessary airfare or hotels). In the United States, in 2004, the same procedure ranges in cost from $13,000 up to $20,000 or more.

The Bileopancreatic Diversion with Duodenal Switch (BPD)

In this procedure, about 75 percent of the stomach is removed and discarded, and a precisely measured length of intestine is attached to the remaining stomach. In BPD, two separate stomach entities—one to collect the food and one to make gastric juices—are not created as they are in GBP.

In BPD, most of the original stomach is cut away. The remaining stomach is a reservoir for food and a location for pepsin and acids to begin breaking down proteins. The small intestine is reconnected according to a precise formula that is based on the length of each person's small intestine. (See Illustration 1–5, which shows BPD with DS, on page 20.)

In BPD, stomach contents mix with gastric juices just like they would normally in the smaller remaining stomach "reservoir" that can hold approximately 4 to 6 ounces. The bile and pancreatic juices are mixed farther down in the small intestine at the Y-shaped junction.

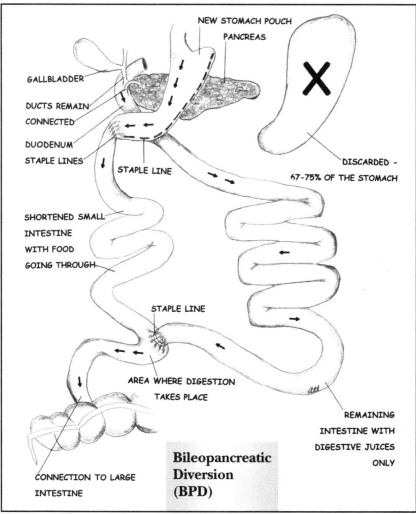

NEW STOMACH POUCH

PANCREAS

GALLBLADDER

DUCTS REMAIN CONNECTED

DUODENUM

STAPLE LINES

STAPLE LINE

DISCARDED - 67-75% OF THE STOMACH

SHORTENED SMALL INTESTINE WITH FOOD GOING THROUGH

STAPLE LINE

AREA WHERE DIGESTION TAKES PLACE

REMAINING INTESTINE WITH DIGESTIVE JUICES ONLY

CONNECTION TO LARGE INTESTINE

Bileopancreatic Diversion (BPD)

Illustration 1-5

This procedure works through malabsorption and restriction. It seems to eliminate intestinal ulcers that are sometimes a problem with gastric bypass. The surgeon usually removes the appendix to prevent inflammation, and the gallbladder to prevent the formation of gallstones. The stomach eventually stretches, allowing the patient to eat at near normal levels with decreased absorption of the fat because the pancreatic juices are not mixed with the partially digested stomach contents until just before the connection to the large intestine. There is a possibility of greater weight loss and maintenance of weight loss. The malabsorption of fat helps prevent those who overindulge on fatty foods from regaining weight.

Although it is extremely rare, and may also be a result of having poor anal sphincter control before surgery, a handful of patients may also experience fecal incontinence because of the poorly digested fat and consistency of the waste materials.

The BPD with *Duodenal Switch (DS) is* a variation of the procedure that preserves the stomach-to-small intestine opening (pyloric valve) and a portion of the first 1 to 2 inches of the small intestine (duodenum). Its proponents say it prevents some potential malnutrition complications of BPD. Nowadays, the BPD is almost always done with a DS to prevent complications.

The Bileopancreatic Diversion causes weight loss primarily by impairing the absorption of certain foods, namely fats and starches, as well as some vitamins and minerals. There is some decrease in the capacity to eat, caused by reduction in the size of the stomach. Rearrangement of the bowel, with a short segment of "common channel," causes most of the fat to be wasted, and 75 to 80 percent of starch, as well.

Patients can eat fairly normal meals, and absorb only a small fraction of the total calories that pass through their mouths. Most persons who are hearty eaters are captivated by the fact that they can continue to eat relatively large amounts.

Superficially this may seem to be a great solution, but it is an illusion. The physiology of digestion and absorption of the many nutrients we need is a very complex process, of which we really understand very little. Our stomachs may have evolved to be a certain size for a reason. Surgical tinkering with this complex process is a bit like letting a five-year-old pull parts out of the back of a color TV. The downside and risks are considerable:

- Protein malnutrition occurs in up to 10 percent of patients, and may require revision (not reversal).
- Absorption of essential vitamins and minerals such as calcium, iron, vitamins A, D, and E is seriously impaired in nearly 100 percent of patients.
- Metabolic bone disease is quite common.
- Bizarre effects on overall metabolism occur, causing strange halitosis, body odors, and a pasty pallor in many patients.
- Wasted starches that are eliminated in the colon (large intestine) lead to production of severely foul-smelling gas, which can be a serious social problem.
- Wasted fats that are passed to the colon are acted upon by bacteria and produce irritating by-products that cause irritable and explosive bowel activity.
- Patients can still regain weight, or fail to lose it, by eating too many foods containing simple sugars or carbohydrates.
- Patients expend a considerable amount of energy and effort seeking solutions to avoid these side effects and inconveniences.[10]

Jejuno-Ileal Bypass (JIB)

This is the operation many physicians and patients think about when bariatric surgery is being discussed. It consisted of stomach stapling and skipping most of the small intestines. All that was left, out of the 20 or so feet of small bowel, was one or two feet, in which digestion could occur. The detached small bowel was left floating inside the person's abdomen in case the patient ever needed a reversal, but it was non-functioning.

Developed in the 1950s, this procedure was the first surgical therapy for morbid obesity. This operation became *very* common in the mid to late 1970s because it was technically easy to perform, it led to large substantial weight loss, and it required minimal effort on the part of the patients. Unfortunately, years after the operation, many patients developed kidney or liver disease and some died as a delayed result of the operation. The JIB is no longer performed because of the preponderance of negative outcomes.

Implantable Gastric Stimulation System (IGS)

In this surgery, a battery pack is implanted under the skin, and a wire that provides electrical stimulation is extended from it to the stomach. The implanted electronic wire leads to the vagus

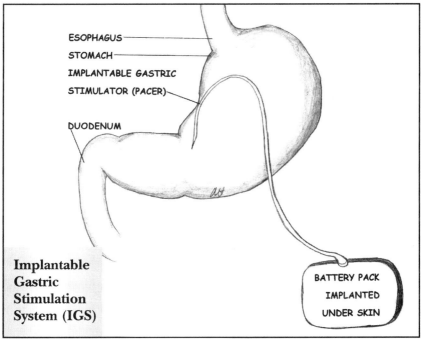

ESOPHAGUS
STOMACH
IMPLANTABLE GASTRIC
STIMULATOR (PACER)
DUODENUM

Implantable Gastric Stimulation System (IGS)

BATTERY PACK
IMPLANTED
UNDER SKIN

Illustration 1-6

nerve of the stomach; when electrical impulses are applied to it, it causes a slowing of the natural movement (peristalsis) of food from the stomach to the small bowel. This is supposed to make the patient feel "full" and lower food intake. The battery pack, very similar to a heart pacemaker, lies just below the skin and can be programmed by a device which lays on top of the skin. Different amounts and frequencies of electrical stimulation are being tested to discover which would prove the most effective in controlling appetite. Currently, the surgeon turns up the electrical current to the point where the patient feels nauseous, then turns it down a bit so the patient just feels "not hungry." This is a new procedure that the FDA is testing in 10 hospitals across the United States, and that may be available in 1 to 2 years. It is available in Europe. (See Illustration 1–6 on page 23.)

First tested in pigs, the IGS caused a decrease in eating and body weight without any complications and no mortality. This device does not look quite as promising in terms of *major* weight loss, but may have an important role when other procedures have failed, or when expected weight loss is less than 100 pounds. The major drawbacks to the system are that the batteries need to be changed, and minor surgery is required to allow the doctor to access the implanted electronic box.[11]

The Gastric Balloon

The gastric balloon is placed endoscopically through the esophagus and inflated with saline water once inside the stomach. The balloon thus partially fills up the stomach, giving the patient the feeling of fullness.[12] The balloon moves as the person sits or lies down allowing food to eventually pass out of the stomach. After the treatment, usually 6 months, the balloon is deflated and

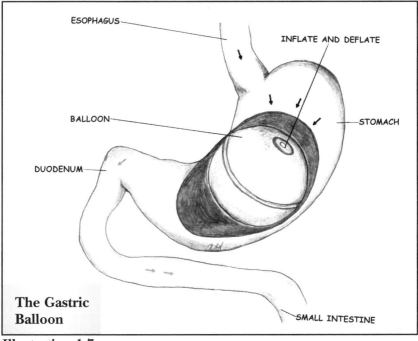

ESOPHAGUS

INFLATE AND DEFLATE

BALLOON

STOMACH

DUODENUM

The Gastric Balloon

SMALL INTESTINE

Illustration 1-7

removed through the esophagus. The procedure is primarily intended for patients who don't have a huge amount of weight to lose. However, the real test is keeping weight off once it's been lost.

Mortality Rates for Bariatric Patients

A survey of mortality among weight loss surgery patients was, and is, being conducted by Dr. Edward Mason of the University of Iowa. He found that, according to the National Death Index, 107 of the 2,363 men studied between 1986 and 1998 died. A regression analysis shows that weight, age, body mass index, history of heart disease, and a history of kidney disease were significant predictors of 30-day post-operative mortality. Twelve addition variables, including whether a simple restrictive operation or a bypass procedure was performed, were not significant predictors.[13]

Here is the mortality timetable:

Within 30 days	17
One to six months	8
One year (+ 6 months)	9
Two to five years (+ 6 months)	32
Six to ten years (+ 6 months)	32
Greater than 10 years	9
Total	**107**

(Reproduced with permission from *Obesity Surgery*)

The 10-year mortality rate, according to this study, is 4.5 percent for bariatric surgery. Most surgical mortality rates are reported for only the first 30 days after the surgery.[14] The 0.5 to 1 percent mortality rate usually recited for bariatric surgery comes from this standard of reporting deaths within the first 30 days.

The mortality rate for the general male population during this same time was approximately 120 deaths for the same number of people. This is about 5.3 percent, or slightly higher than for those undergoing bariatric surgery. Bariatric surgery seems to be effective in at least reducing slightly the mortality rate slightly over time. More studies are needed to confirm this finding.

How Big is the Mature Pouch?

All of the procedures discussed leave patients with a small stomach pouch. As the months pass, it will enlarge somewhat. Some of this is actual enlargement, and some is due to a softening of the pouch and its outlet. The cottage cheese test is a technique that was presented at the June 2000 meeting of the American Society for Bariatric Surgery (ASBS) by Latham Flanagan, MD. It is meant to be a standardized, reproducible measurement of the size of the stomach pouch.

1. Purchase a 16-ounce container of small-curd low-fat cottage cheese. Begin the test with a full container, and perform the test in the morning before eating anything else (this will be your breakfast on that day). Eat fairly quickly until you feel full (less than five minutes). Note that the small soft curds do not require much chewing. The idea with the rapid eating is to fill the pouch before there is much time for food to flow out of it.

2. After eating your fill of cottage cheese, you will be left with a partially eaten container that has empty space where cottage cheese used to be.

3. Start with a measured amount of water (16 ounces, for example), and pour water into the container of cottage cheese until the water is level with the original top level of the cottage cheese.

The amount of water poured into the container is the functional size of the pouch.

If this is your first time doing the test, don't panic. You are likely to find that the size of your pouch is bigger than your surgeon told you she made it at the time of surgery. Dr. Flanagan's data indicates that the average size of the mature pouch measured by this test is 5.5 ounces. He has also found that sizes ranging from 3 to 9 ounces have no impact on the person's success in weight loss.[15]

Summary

Which surgical procedure is the best? To answer that question, several factors must be considered:

* *How much weight does the person have to lose?*

A simple restrictive banding (the VBG or AGB) may not produce desired results for a person who has well over 100 pounds to lose.

* *How compliant will the patient be to doctor's instructions?*

To thrive after a complex procedure such as the GBP or BPD, the person *must* adhere to a rigorous daily supplement schedule.

* *Is the patient ill to begin with?*

A more complex surgery (GBP or BPD) may result in a higher incidence of complications in those who are already ill.

* *How amenable is the patient to sticking with a diet while losing the weight?*

The AGB and VBG require that you be put on a diet to lose weight because all food eaten is converted to energy or fat. With the GBP or BPD, some calories, mainly fats and starches, are wasted. Therefore, the food must be highly nutritious—not just junk food.

* *How much, in terms of side effects, is the person willing to tolerate?*

The BPD will produce the most significant weight loss with the least restrictive regimen. However, potential side effects are major and may be disabling.

- *Is the person likely to follow a rigorous change in eating habits?*

People who do not comply with the nutrition regimen pre-scribed by their doctor are likely to become malnourished. If the patient does not plan to consume protein drinks and extra vita-mins and minerals, the only possible positive outcomes would result from the proximal GBP, the AGB, or the VBG.

- *Is the person able to stop consuming sweets?*

This has been a problem with adult-onset diabetics who do not care to stop eating sweets and sugar-based foods. If the person is not able to stop, the GBP operations would not be a good choice for him or her.

- *Is the person willing and able to pay $100 to $150 a month for the supplements they are required to take?*

These are not covered by insurance, but their price will be offset by the minimal amount of food consumed.

People who are rebellious may defy doctor's orders, thinking they can lose weight no matter what they eat. This is true; with bypass surgery, patients can lose weight while eating candy bars and doughnuts. However, their chances of health and survival aren't very good due to the malnutrition patients will suffer from eating such a diet. Such a person might be better off using weight-control drugs and waiting for the IGS system or a hunger-blocking pill to become available.

For people with fewer than 100 pounds to lose who want to avail themselves of a weight loss device, the gastric balloon has been refined and is showing promise as an adjunct to weight loss. But once the balloon is removed from the stomach, it's necessary to alter eating habits and exercise patterns to offset weight gain.

The physician who is familiar with all types of bariatric surgeries would most likely be the person to help with the decision about which procedure to have. However, some doctors gravitate toward certain surgeries and others are competent with all types. Research and explore the many kinds of surgeries available so that you have a wide knowledge base. In this way, you will not only be fully informed of risks and expectations, but you will also be in a better position to comply with the lifestyle changes necessary to ensure long-term success after your chosen procedure.

2

What Changing Your Body Image May Mean

A power inside you waits to be released. All of the potential psychological problems associated with losing over half your body fat can be dealt with when you are committed to becoming healthy in all aspects of your life.

Until one is committed, there is hesitancy. The horror stories you will hear from people who know the aunt of a friend who had weight loss surgery 30 years ago, with negative results, may convince you to resist making a decision. But, once you have decided to proceed with the surgery, you will notice that this commitment alone will initiate changes within. It is also important to be sure that the center in which you choose to have your surgery has support groups to help you deal with the consequences resulting from the procedure. It is wise to attend a support group before surgery.

There is risk associated with these procedures, but they are safer now than they were in the past. Ask your doctor about the number of procedures he has performed and the mortality and serious side effect rates associated with the procedures. Ask the nurses in the center where your doctor works if he is competent. They know more than anyone on the doctor's paid staff about what results can be expected. Empower yourself—be informed.

Are you so unhappy with yourself that you would rather die than continue with the body you have? Putting your fate in the hands of the surgeon does carry that immediate risk. The risk of mortality is 1 in 150 during the first 30 days after surgery and 7 in 150 over the next 10 years.[1]

If you decide to go ahead with one of the procedures described in this book, there is an excellent reference by Bryan G. Woodward, titled *The Complete Guide to Obesity Surgery.*[2] His book is definitely pro-surgery and assumes that the person reading it has already decided to proceed with the operation. It will take you through all the steps from pre- to post-surgery. This book is a must-read for anyone who has positively decided to have this surgery.

Body Types

There are things in your life that you have always accepted as being unchangeable, such as your height, eye color, or shoe size. Despite feeling discouraged by countless failed diets and regaining of lost pounds, you have also suspected that your body type was ultimately beyond your control. You were right: body type is, indeed, inherited.

Within certain parameters, we are given an ectomorphic (skinny), mesomorphic (average) or endomorphic (heavy) body type.[3] An ectomorph will never be fat. This is the person who, while growing up, is called derogatory names such as "bean pole," or "anorexic" because they are so thin. They usually remain thin through child-bearing years and into their fifties without effort. Their arms and legs remain thin but some may eventually gain 10 to 20 pounds with age and get a slight potbelly. They don't look muscular, even when they work out. They never have to worry about being fat and almost never think about going on a diet to control their weight.

Mesomorphs are of normal weight during childhood and adolescence. They are often muscular and athletic-looking in their youth. If female, they may begin to put on a little additional weight with each pregnancy and if they aren't vigilant about taking it off, it may be there to stay. Men who have sedentary jobs may have to work out religiously as they get older. In their fifties, these people may be 20 to 50 pounds over their ideal weight and must watch what they eat. They may look large, but don't have the rounded, non-muscular body that is typical of endomorphs.

Endomorphs are those people who were heavy as children and adolescents. Their arms and legs have a rounded, ill-defined, non-muscular appearance. If female, they remain heavy and put on weight with each succeeding pregnancy. If they are male, they may be able to control their weight with heavy manual labor. However, once they become more sedentary, the weight piles on without any eating changes. They are eventually 100 or more pounds overweight despite repeated major attempts at losing weight. They are the "super absorbers," a term we'll discuss in Chapter 8. They may be genetically predisposed toward runaway weight-gain, despite dieting attempts. They never seem to feel full, even after consuming enormous amounts of food. Certain drugs, such as Phentermine Fenfluramine (Fen-Phen or Phen-Fen, no longer available) and others, may have helped them control hunger in the past, but their effectiveness eventually diminished and weight was regained.

Throughout history, body types have been associated with certain personality types. The ectomorph (skinny) person is seen as being restrained, inhibited and very private. The mesomorph (average) person is thought to be sturdy, vigorous, energetic and assertive, and the endomorph (heavy) person is thought of as sociable, friendly, relaxed and unmotivated. These stereotypes continue today.

Whether or not people are as healthy and fit as they could be, within the boundaries of their given body type, remains an individual decision about diet and exercise. All three groups can be physically fit and healthy, even though they may weigh more or less than the weight tables allow. There are some endomorphs who are fit enough to run marathons and even participate in the iron-man competition. But they do so at a significantly higher weight than the mesomorphs. It is more essential, with respect to longevity, to be fit than to be lean. A fat person who is fit will generally live longer than a lean person who is unfit.

You can't change your body type without artificially altering your food intake or energy output to such a significant degree that the "natural" weight is not sustainable. Surgery to control food intake and/or food absorption is the only known external control that seems to work for the morbidly obese. After surgery, daily food intake is reduced to less than is normally consumed in one meal. Because absorption of nutrients is so altered, supplements are required to prevent malnutrition-related diseases.

Metropolitan Insurance Company Weight Tables

The Metropolitan Insurance Company first issued its height-weight tables in 1897, in an attempt to indicate the lowest mortality rates, so that they could charge higher premiums for those who didn't fit within their parameters. The first weight tables took into account the age of the individual. For example, a women who was 5 feet 4 inches tall could weigh:

126 pounds between ages 20 and 29
132 pounds between ages 30 and 39
140 pounds between ages 40 and 49
145 pounds between ages 50 and 59
144 pounds between ages 60 and 69.

Originally, the tables did not provide ranges for small, average, or large frames—they were added later, although never defined. A person was not thought to be at risk until 20 percent over or under what the weight tables allowed. That first attempt at defining an average weight is what seems to have gotten the fat-conscious psyche going.

In 1942, new tables were published that no longer indicated differing weights for separate age groups. These new tables contained suggested weights for small, medium, or large frames, although instructions about how to determine the size of one's frame were never provided. The label designation also contained a major change. It no longer read "average" weight, but "ideal" weight, suggesting that it was not okay to gain weight with age. Even though this idea may be erroneous, it has stayed with us and survived. Nowadays, there is scarcely an issue of a health or woman's magazine that does not address weight control in some way.

In 1959, the Metropolitan height-weight tables were again revised. The suggested weights were lowered and referred to as "desirable" rather than "average" or "ideal." The tables were changed mainly because people were larger than ever before and the insurance companies assumed that increases in weight would lead to increases in mortality—a theory based on conjecture rather than fact.

When the height-weight tables were again revised in 1983 by the Metropolitan Insurance Company, the new standards were unequivocally heavier than those in 1959. Short men and women benefited the most from this change, and could weigh 10 to 13 pounds more than in previous years. Men and women of medium or tall height could weigh an additional two to eight pounds. A scientific survey called the Build Study[4] indicated the best weights for longevity had increased by amounts up to 17 percent over those that had been recommended for the previous generation. This study found that body weights associated with lowest mortality increased progressively with age. However, the Metropolitan charts don't reflect that finding.

The Body Mass Index (BMI) [See Chapter 9.] is a ratio of fat to lean body tissue. There is pressure by health professionals to set the ideal BMI for males at around 15 and for females at around 22. However, by the time a woman reaches her sixties, for example, the BMI associated with lowest mortality is found to be 27.3—in other words, clinically obese. In fact, women with the lowest mortality rates were older, between 5 feet 2 and 5 feet 4 inches tall, with weights ranging from 180 to 190 pounds. The Build Study seemed to indicate that the ideal weights represented by the Metropolitan Insurance Company charts for many years have been misleading people who rely on that data as being scientifically correct.[5]

Shifting the Way You Think about Food

If you elect to have weight loss surgery you will begin thinking about weight in a new way. After the surgery, your body type will *seem* to be one of the first two types, ectomorph or mesomorph—but no longer endomorphic. Your mind-set, however, will remain that of an endomorph.

There is evidence that a hunger enzyme called ghrelin and others may be reduced with bypass surgery, significantly altering perceived hunger levels. You will need to come to a new understanding with your body and mind. Creating the "new you" will involve giving up some of the things you have previously enjoyed: large meals, chips, sweets, and candy. And you will have to adjust to different bowel habits, frequent loose stools, possible constipation, and for most, excess malodorous gas.

These changes must be felt, acknowledged and in some cases mourned and let go. The guilt, anger, and grief over your body size will also disappear. In its place will be feelings of pride, satisfaction, and love of your physical self. Keep in mind that self-hatred related to dissatisfaction with your personality or other aspects of your life will not change with surgery.

Somatoform Personality Types

Some people grow up in an environment of ill health. Being ill has its rewards for such people: They get the attention of a parent or spouse. They get to feel sorry for themselves and believe they have a reason to be unhappy. They can be alone and aloof and not be blamed because they are sick. There are even many people who use illness as an escape from facing up to themselves. Sometimes these people are so wrapped up in their physical selves that they remain unaware of their own feelings.

People with a somatoform personality translate frightening, angry feelings into physical complaints. They may get a rash because they feel ashamed. They may get a headache because they cheated on their taxes or told a lie. They may come down with a tickle in their throat because they said something they wish they had not, or they may get a stomachache before a meeting with their boss. Often, being fat serves an important role in their lives. They can make excuses for unacceptable behavior because they do not feel great about themselves. Somehow, other folks should understand. They can refuse to feel the anger and hurt that accompany snide remarks and sometimes learn to seek comfort in the very thing that is the cause of those remarks—excessive eating.

"Stuffing anger" is another common defense mechanism among obese people. Instead of confronting the source of the anger—be it another person or their own feelings about the anger—the person overeats to ease his or her discomfort. Eating too much makes it possible for them to tune out the world. Nothing feels as good as the food going in, and no drug is as powerful as the mindless haze in which they find themselves after a binge. There is a physical basis for this. The feel-good hormone dopamine is released into the bloodstream as we chew, smell, and swallow. Serotonin is then released as the food is digested. After bingeing, a person forgets the hurt, anger, disappointment, or frustration that triggered the binge. Relief and forgetting begin with the very first bite. The focus changes from inner feelings to food, and how good it tastes and feels. These people are taking care of themselves in the only way they know how to—with food. They need to develop new methods of coping with the negative aspects of life if they undergo weight loss surgery.

Surgical Remedies and their Consequences

Why would anyone want to have weight loss surgery? It involves giving up eating normally for the rest of your life. You can never "go off it" as you can with dieting. It is permanent and can be reversed only with very serious consequences and expense. You have to adhere to a strict regimen of supplements and protein drinks every day of your life to offset the constant threat of malnutrition. The large meals that you indulge in at restaurants and home will no longer be an option; you will throw up several times if you eat large quantities. You will now be eating meals that could fit in a shot glass. However, because your stomach is so small, you will allegedly not be hungry. With some of the surgeries, this may be partially true; with others that do not alter the stomach in any way (such as the VBG and AGB), hunger levels remain as they were before the surgery.

Surgical remedies are the most extreme measures you can take to control your weight, and present the most risks. Within a few years there may be gene therapy or a drug that will make these procedures obsolete but, until then, this is the only method of weight control that works. Other weight loss programs have a success rate of 3 percent.[6] Any disease or condition that has a 97 percent failure rate is essentially incurable.

For years, you thought that if you could just control your eating, if you could just stay on the program that you selected, you could be thin. The media—magazine articles, books, TV ads for prescription drugs—and friends, parents, spouses, even doctors sent messages that your weight was your fault. If *you* could just change, you would be a normal-weight person.

If you've always been overweight, your problems may not be your fault. Body type is 70 percent or more genetic. You are genetically programmed to weigh a certain amount, or within a certain range, depending on your activity level. This is as much a part of your heritage as your eye color, height, hand size, and nose shape.

These other characteristics do not affect your self-esteem in the same way your weight does. In the 1950s, the average model weighed 8 percent less than the average woman. That means that an average-sized woman, who weighed 145 pounds, saw women in the media who weighed about 135 pounds. By the 1990s, the average model and actress weighed 25 percent less than the average woman. That means if an average woman weighed 145 pounds, she was comparing herself to models and actresses who weighed about 109 pounds—the ultimate "ideal women".[7] Keep in mind that today the average size of women's pants sold in America is 16. Such discrepancies between "real" and "ideal" help set the stage for the current epidemic of eating disorders, low self-esteem, depression, "put-downs," and feelings of guilt and shame.

Prejudice against Fat People

Insulting those who are overweight is the last acceptable form of discrimination. In an article titled, "The Problem of Obesity," medical writer Faith Fitzgerald says:

> *It is clear from reading magazines or watching television that the public derision and condemnation of fat people is one of the few remaining sanctioned social prejudices in this nation freely allowed against any group based solely on appearance.[8]*

Health and nutrition writer Lew Louderback[9] puts into words the general view that is shared by many about being overweight:

> *Everything from idle comment to the repetitive hammering of the mass media confirms the message: fat is ugly. It is self-indulgent, therefore immoral. It is certainly un-American, for the President's Counsel on Physical Fitness has declared war on it in no uncertain terms. Fat is sick...overweight individuals*

eat to assuage their feelings of inferiority, insecurity, sexual
inadequacy. Fat is unhealthy, in fact suicidal. Actuarial tables
are there to show us that each extra pound of flesh is another
nail in our coffins.

What Louderback says is supported by tracking the socioeconomic changes in obesity, originally associated with lower
socioeconomic status. Women of lower socioeconomic status
were six times more likely to be obese than women of upper
socioeconomic status. By six years of age, obesity was nine times
more prevalent in girls of lower economic status than girls who
were wealthy. However, as the ease and availability of high-fat
foods has increased, and children are left unsupervised for a
portion of the day, all socioeconomic groups have been gravitat-
ing toward snack foods that are high in fat and sugar because
they require little or no effort to prepare. As the number of one-
parent homes increases, wealthy obese children are quickly
catching up to the poor.[10]

Even fat people seem to have a problem with people who
are fatter than they are. We tend to regard the fat person as
slow, lazy, and as having no self-control. Unfortunately, this is
accepted as truth when, in fact, it is often inaccurate. There is
no one so self-controlled as the person who has stayed on a
diet and exercise program and lost 50 to 100 pounds, sometimes more than once. There is no one more committed to
exercise than the fat person who has gotten into shorts or a
swimsuit day after day and who has gone to the gym or on a
walk to lose weight, despite severe joint pain, ridicule, and dis-
approving looks. There is no one so quick of mind as the fat
person who hears another veiled put-down and decides how
much to let it affect them. Fat people are anything but slow,
lazy and without control, but the morbidly obese are in a no-

win situation—the only reliable cure for their condition at present is weight loss surgery.

Even doctors who deal with obese people may have a bias against overweight individuals. The old stereotypes still exist: lower social standing, laziness, diminished feelings and intelligence. In one survey, doctors with the least amount of weight bias were older males who had a positive mental outlook, weighed more, and had friends who were obese.[11]

Emotional Considerations

It is almost impossible to describe the range of emotions that one goes through when deciding to have this surgery. It is almost like committing to die on a certain day. In some ways, your old life will be gone. Your relationship with food will change dramatically. Eating for comfort, eating to "stuff" feelings, eating to fill loneliness, will no longer be viable options.

Food means much more than nourishment for most of us. We all use food for reasons other than hunger. Once you have this surgery, you will have to relate to food differently. You will quickly discover, through unintended vomiting or The Dumping Syndrome (see page 11), that eating too much can be very unpleasant. Heartburn and pain will result from overeating, and a meal may be one-quarter to one-half a cup or less.

In some ways, the emotions that led you to overeat in the past will be replaced by feelings of success as your weight comes off. You will begin to get positive feedback from many people. You will suddenly be seen as smart and active—someone in command of the situation. People will treat you differently. It may be difficult to remember that losing weight through forced mini-meals is not really anything you control. It happens because your stomach is now the size of a golf ball. Many women begin to take better care of their skin, hair, nails and clothes. Men are suddenly enthusiastic about going shopping for clothes. Almost all weight loss surgery patients become the people they wanted to look like, but could not because of previous inability to lose weight.

Women who may have been abused in the past may experience great fear when they start to lose weight. Issues of being too pretty or too desirable may surface, and the person may subconsciously sabotage their weight loss by drinking high-calorie drinks, or by not following their nutrition regimen. In a famous study cited in the book, *Awakening Intuition* by Mona Lisa Schulz, rats were raised in boxes where, from birth, they regularly received electric shocks.[12] It sounds awful, but for the rats it was home sweet home. It is not unlike that for many people who grow up with great trauma. Once the rats reached adulthood, they were allowed to leave their original boxes and move to others in which no shocks were administered. The rats chose to return to their original homes and to life amid the shocks. Thus, the rats demonstrated a preference for reliving their known distress, rather than opting for an unknown, more comfortable future.

In the same way, many people grow accustomed to lives where they were ridiculed and lonely. It's familiar. The prospects of being good-looking, or trying to make and keep friends, or having men or women pay attention to them, are threatening. These people need to look closely at their reasons for wanting to drastically change their body shape. Health and disease prevention may be enough of a reason to go ahead. If someone is truly driven by a death wish, however, perhaps such a drastic change will have deleterious effects. They may become depressed if they lose weight and their life problems do not magically disappear. If they successfully lose weight, they will no longer have something to blame—and looking inward may be painful.

Controlling Thoughts and Feelings

It is not what happened to us in the past that causes our problems—our memories and associated meanings are what continue to haunt us. We can erase negative memories from our lives by giving them less and less attention. Almost all the cells in our bodies have been changed and renewed since a traumatic childhood event. We are new people with old thoughts. Gradually let the old thoughts go because, as long as we have acknowledged the feelings around these incidents and changed what we can, we can also acknowledge that it was not our fault, and forget it. Memories that are not constantly relived will fade with time and become less important. A person who has kept a vile memory or experience alive for decades, with the physical manifestation of that trauma being their weight, feels threatened when they become thin. These people will need psychiatric support following surgery. Philosopher C. Terry Warner a says:

> *The only change that matters is a change of heart. Every other change alters us cosmetically but not fundamentally, modifies how we appear or what we do, but not who we are. Our hearts change when resentment, anxiety, and self-worry give way to openness, sensitivity and love of life[13]*

Positive Aspects of Weight-Loss Surgery

Most people who have weight loss surgery have generally positive results, and the negatives are greatly over-shadowed by the thrill of finally being thin. For most people, there are few regrets.

Some even say that they would go through the surgery every month if necessary in order to stay thin. Being thin is so important in our society that, when a person who has been 100 pounds or more overweight finally becomes thin, he or she feels on top of the world. They have won the jackpot, and a million dollars would not tempt them to go back to the way they were.

They may actually become new people, with new thoughts, an active lifestyle, and more self-esteem. They have become the people they always wanted to be, but were not allowed to be, because of the fat on their bodies. The positive new thoughts they now experience have caused a biochemical response by increasing their endorphin levels. The thoughts we hold on to long enough eventually become our reality. As TV psychologist Dr. Phil McGraw says, we make our own reality through our thoughts and actions.[14]

A dramatic adjustment of your entire system of beliefs is required to go from thinking "I am fat" to "I am thin." In the book, *Women's Bodies, Women's Wisdom,*[15] there is an experiment in which Dr. Ellen Languer studied a group of male volunteers over the age of 70 at a five-day retreat. The men all agreed that they would live in the present as though it were 1959. They would let themselves be who they had been at that time. They brought in pictures of themselves from that year and put them around the center. Then their parameters of physical strength, perception, cognition, taste and hearing were measured. Over the course of the five days, many of the parameters, such as hearing and memory, improved. Serial photographs showed that the men looked years younger as well. As they changed their mindsets about aging, in just five days, their physical bodies changed as well.

The regular and irreversible cycles of aging may be partly a product of certain assumptions about how one is supposed to grow old. If we do not feel compelled to carry out these limiting mind-sets, we might have a greater chance of replacing years of decline with years of growth and purpose. In the same way, some people who find themselves thin after years of being fat, create new perceptions for themselves. They feel younger, some of their illnesses and complaints have disappeared and they are more active. Some report feeling younger, and indeed appear younger than they have in years.[16] It is amazing to find out the ages of some of those who have had this surgery. In many cases, after surgery and subsequent weight loss, they appear to have found the Fountain of Youth.

3

Negative Aspects of Weight Loss Surgery

Gastric Bypass Surgery had come under criticism for long-term side effects even before it was first approved by the National Institute of Health (NIH) in December, 1978. As a result of recommendations by the consensus panel working on the problem at the NIH, intestinal bypass was ultimately accepted for health insurance coverage and given a code, thus making thousands of these operations possible. Some insurance policies, however, still specifically exclude these procedures. And observers report that, of the hundreds of thousands of patients worldwide who have had the surgery, most suffer severe complications relating to their digestive health. In addition, questionable advertising has been associated with weight loss surgery. A recent mailing read as follows:

The Mini Gastric Bypass
• No Dieting Ever
• Lose Weight Automatically
• Shed Excess Pounds Fast

- No Exercise Needed
- Never Feel Deprived
- 200 percent More Energy
- 100 percent Safe if Supplements are Properly Taken

These claims are untrue. Dr. E. Patchen Dellinger, a bariatric physician at the University of Washington, has found that "when a person hits 400-plus pounds, even with gastric bypass surgery, dietary modifications, and exercise, it is unlikely that normal weight will ever be achieved." He goes on to say that, "This operation does not cause weight loss. Diet and exercise cause weight loss and the operation assists dieting."[1] The following statements more realistically represent the risks of weight loss surgery:

- I know I have a 1 percent chance of dying within the first 30 days.
- I know that to lose a lot of weight, I will be making a healthy digestive tract, unhealthy.
- I know that I may not lose more than 100 pounds because of genetics.
- I know that even the most drastic intestinal bypass may stop working sometime within 7 years of surgery, and I will have to diet and exercise. But it may be more difficult because my metabolism will have been damaged.
- I know I may suffer complications requiring more surgery, some of them extremely painful, like bowel obstruction.
- I know that losing 100 pounds rapidly puts me at risk for sudden heart attack.
- I know I may get very sick with this surgery no matter what I do.
- I know that any surgery is a tool and that I will have to diet and exercise to keep the weight off.

- I know that, because of risks of malnutrition, I will no longer be able to eat foods that don't contribute to my nutritional needs. This includes all forms of pastry, cookies, chips, ice cream, cakes, and other junk foods. The food I eat should be limited primarily to complex carbohydrates and proteins, including protein drinks made without sugar.

These are the real risks of surgery that people should be aware of in order to make an informed decision.

Nearly every surgical operation originates in a laboratory, where it is refined by extensive tests on animals. For example, coronary bypass surgery was the product of years of experimentation on dogs, in which repeated measurements and detailed autopsies revealed potential complications and allowed surgeons to perfect the procedure. By contrast, only three animal tests have been reported in gastroplasty. A 2003 *Journal of the American Medical Association* article about weight loss surgery stated that the long-term consequences remain uncertain, and the long-term effects of altering nutrient absorption remain unresolved.[2]

The number and variety of bypass operations presents further difficulty. As many as two dozen basic types of gastroplasty and bypass are in current use, along with several modifications. Operations that impair the absorption and processing of nutrients should produce the greatest weight loss, and be most likely to produce lasting weight loss. In one study of vertical banded gastroplasty (VBG), only 24 percent of the patients had maintained their total post-operative weight loss for 30 months; 22 percent had suffered from obstruction of the narrow outlet from the stomach pouch.[3] (for more information about VBG see page 3).

Weight-regain after gastroplasty is usually the result of both the gradual stretching and enlargement of the stomach pouch or the narrow outlet, and the adaptations of the body. Because the stomach can expand, it adapts to increased pressure by becoming less elastic and bigger, like a stretched out balloon. The operation is thus doomed to be at least partially undone by the natural adaptive processes of the patient's body. A person will usually lose all the weight they are going to lose within 12 to 24 months after the surgery. Then, the body adapts and dieting is required, just as it was before the surgery.

Gastric bypass (GBP) is effective for maintaining weight loss, but there are also more long-term complications—particularly nutritional deficiencies—including anemia, pernicious anemia, lupus, osteoporosis, and neurological damage. In addition, autoimmune disorders after surgery may be caused by afferent limb syndrome, in which the unused portion of the intestine develops an overgrowth of bacteria.[4] Without the normal flushing of this leg of the intestine (as would occur with the passage of food and liquids), it tends to play host to a number of unwanted bacteria.

The stomach is not simply a passive sac for storing food, but plays a complex role in the processing of nutrients as well. So, surgical procedures that interfere with its operation can trigger multiple problems. Unfortunately, objective controlled trials that include physical examinations of patients, conducted by doctors not associated with this surgical technique, are rare.

In one instance of independent examination of patients who had received either VGB or GBP surgery, 5 percent were found to have neurological complications (nerve or brain damage)[5] The patients were examined within a year after surgery, so the incidence of long-term neurological deterioration could eventually become much higher.

Normally, once a surgical technique has been developed in the animal laboratory, the next step is to run controlled clinical trials comparing long-term outcomes for patients to those of an untreated control group. Coronary bypass was tested in this way, and it was proven that heart patients undergoing surgery lived longer than comparable patients receiving only nonsurgical treatment. With the exception of one Danish trial of gastric bypass showing that patients undergoing surgery experienced more health problems than comparable patients who were put on low-calorie diets,[6] no such clinical trials have been conducted for weight loss surgery.

Gastric bypass, *does* result in improved levels of blood pressure, cholesterol, and blood sugar. These reduced risk factors might translate into long-term disease prevention if weight loss can be maintained throughout the patient's life span.[7]

Do the benefits of weight loss exceed the risks of major surgery and the side effects of tampering with the digestive system? Is a 50 percent weight loss adequate reason to go ahead with the procedure? We must first consider how long the weight loss can be maintained. Some doctors suggest that, in the least radical procedure, VBG, patients may expect to maintain only a 50 percent loss when weighed five years after surgery. That means that, if you have 100 pounds to lose, you will likely maintain only a 50-pound weight loss five years later—in the interim, you may have lost the original 100 pounds and regained half of it. In such cases, the doctor will sometimes recommend a liquid protein drink diet or a modified fast, much like the Optifast system used by Oprah Winfrey. Unfortunately, that approach does not teach "pouch use," and is detrimental to the patient's already compromised metabolism.

Nutritionists studying weight suspect that many fat people are burdened with a gene, or a combination of genes, that allow renegade weight gain. The Navajo Indians have been studied as one group of "super-absorbers," with a genetic tendency to gain weight. Many people also have what has been termed a "thrifty gene"—a gene, or set of genes, that tend to hold onto fat stores.[8] They are severely at risk for weight-related diseases. One theory suggests that some of the eight weight-related genes that have been identified "turn on" at different times. If you get one of the genes, you may experience renegade weight gain in childhood, another may turn on in adolescence, another with pregnancy, and another in middle age. Some of the genes are related to age and others are related to overall metabolism. If you get all eight (identified so far) genes associated with obesity, you are assured of having problems with weight gain unless exercise levels are so high that you don't store excess fat—an unlikely scenario in our modern day.

Operating on obese patients is riskier than operating on slender people for many reasons. To begin with, they do not breathe well, and present many weight-related complications during, and after, surgery. Because fat absorbs drugs and anesthetic gases, much higher doses (which take longer to be eliminated) are required to be effective. And the difficulties of moving an unconscious patient are compounded when that patient weighs 400 or more pounds. Dr. Dellinger points out that accommodations have to be made to properly care for obese patients. "Obese patients often can't sit on a hospital toilet without breaking it. They're too heavy to have surgery on a regular operating table because it won't sustain their weight."[9]

Second, during traditional abdominal surgery, internal organs must be separated and held apart to permit the surgeon a clear field of vision. Keeping the obese patient's excess fat from moving and obscuring the surgeon's view during a weight loss procedure presents a challenge. Further, the patient's abdominal wall may be 4 to 5 inches thick; ordinary surgical instruments cannot reach that far, and longer instruments are harder to learn to manipulate precisely. Even X rays do not penetrate as well, and are less clear.[10] Post-surgical complications most commonly include pulmonary embolism, pneumonia, and healing wound infections.

Another issue concerns the anticipated life span of women. Normal-weight women have a life expectancy of around 79 years. Women who are 100 to 150 pounds overweight have a 5-year reduced life expectancy of 74 years. This is equivalent to the life expectancy of a light smoker. But even these extremely obese women still have a longer life expectancy than the 72 years of normal-weight men.

A person who is considering this surgery should evaluate the number of decades they will have to be impaired, and the risks of malnutrition associated with bypass surgery over their entire remaining life span. People with an apple body shape, with more fat around the mid-section, are at greater risk and tend to have more complications with surgery than pear-shaped people who have heavy hips and thighs. Clearly, surgery should be considered only for the most obese patients with a BMI greater than 40 and a 100-pound or more weight problem. Exceptions should be made only if the patient currently suffers from life-threatening disease that may be ameliorated by weight loss surgery. It is essential that the patient acquire all the facts regarding weight loss and complications resulting from the surgery (see Appendix II). The person must be prepared to never eat normally again. Food as a social and pleasurable experience may disappear, and tiny amounts of food with supplements, must become the routine for survival. Instead of internally controlled hunger, the surgical procedure will make satiety (feeling full) impossible for the emotional eater who generally eats to fill the void created by loneliness, deprivation, or fear.

Risks of Malnutrition

There is a distinct possibility that a person will become malnourished following gastric bypass surgery, but steps can be taken to help ensure that this does not happen. One solution is to drink several high-protein shakes every day. The problem with drinking high-protein shakes is that they are not always available, nor do people always feel like having one. The strict vitamin and mineral supplement regimen is also subject to patient compliance.

Malnutrition may also be a factor in healing following surgery. Two major studies have assessed malnutrition in conjunction with slower-healing patterns. One, conducted in 1984, found that malnourished patients have less successful subsequent surgeries of any sort.[11] This study showed 86 percent of patients with normal serum albumen levels healed successfully after surgery, compared to 20 percent with low serum albumin, an indicator of malnutrition. The second, in 1987, reported that 6 percent of well-nourished patients experienced local or systemic complications compared to 44 percent who were malnourished.[12] Few people who have weight loss surgery anticipate that they will eventually need other surgeries for various unrelated reasons. However, the decision to have weight loss surgery may determine the outcome for those later surgeries because of how well-nourished the person is and if undetected damage has been sustained because of weight loss surgery.

Risks of Weight Loss Surgery

Risks of weight loss surgery include any and all of the risks normally associated with any major surgery.

- Allergic reactions ranging from a rash to sudden overwhelming reactions that cause death.
- Anesthetic complications including an overdose, the wrong kind, or an allergic reaction.
- Bleeding (from minor to massive), emergency surgery, or transfusion
- Blood clots (also called deep-vein thrombosis and pulmonary embolus).
- Infection of the wound, bladder infection, pneumonia, skin infections, or deep abdominal infections.
- Leaking of stomach acid, bacteria, and digestive enzymes into the abdominal cavity.
- Ulcers and narrowing at the connection between the stomach and small bowel in 13 to 20 percent of patients.
- Bowel obstruction or blockage.
- Dumping syndrome, which includes heart palpitations, weakness, sweating, nausea, dizziness, diarrhea, and a feeling of impending doom.
- Medication side effects.
- Loss of bodily function including stroke, heart attack, limb loss, and other problems.
- Risk of hepatitis and AIDS from the administration of blood.
- Hernia in the abdominal wall (common in bypass surgeries).
- Hair loss (a frequent short-term complaint).
- Vitamin and mineral deficiencies because of malabsorption. Deficiencies of iron, folate, and B12 have been found in many patients after bypass.
- Complications of pregnancy and risk to the fetus can occur, especially during the first year after the operation.

- Depression, a common medical illness, can be a result of giving up a basic human function—eating normally.
- Many coffee, tea, and caffeinated soda drinkers experience severe headaches following surgery. Caffeine consumption needs to be stopped well ahead of the operation.

The total expected complication rate is about 30 percent, or one in three, for major or minor complications in the weeks immediately following surgery. Some people have both major and minor complications, while others have none at all. The major risks of weight loss surgery are from respiratory failure, blood clots and leakage of stomach contents into the surrounding tissues. Eighty percent of the people who die within the first 30 days after surgery have one of these complications.[13] No known long-term studies have been performed outlining the expected complications over the life span of the individual. One study, currently in its tenth year, indicates that the ten-year mortality rate for bariatric patients is 4.5 percent.[14] No one has found it to be superior for life expectancy, or for anything else other than certain risk factors, compared to more conservative clinical treatment. A few trials have been started, but their final results remain unreported.

Why?

When Dr. Paul Ernsberger appeared on the Donahue show in 2002, he speculated that the reason final results from clinical bariatric trials hadn't been released was because the news was bad. In an April 2003 article, Dr. Edward Livingston stated that such a trial would show that the benefits of surgery have been "overestimated."[15] The U.S. government has provided for such a five-year study (scheduled to begin soon) which, like the Hormone Response (Estrogen) trials, might produce fascinating results.

4

Risks of Obesity

It is no secret that obesity has become a major problem in America. More than 30 percent of Americans are considered obese and 1 in 50 adults weighs is overweight by at least 100 pounds.

Studies of obesity and its associated health risks have approached the subject as a static condition: A person is fat and therefore has certain risk factors. There are, however, many ways to define obesity. The difference between fat people and thin people who are sedentary is minimal, while the difference between a sedentary fat person and a fat person who is fit is significant. People who have dieted, lost weight, and then gained it back multiple times are likely to have more risk factors than those who have never tried dieting. There are those who are aerobically fit but fat, those who are sedentary and fat, and the yo-yo dieters. Studies need to differentiate between these different kinds of obesity in order to be able to state with authority that obesity alone is the causative risk factor for the conditions to be discussed in this chapter.

Cardiovascular Disease and Heart Disease

Obesity has long been thought to be a risk factor for heart disease, high blood pressure, and stroke. One study reported that obesity in childhood is a stronger predictor of heart disease than a family history of the condition.[1]

As we learned in Chapter 2, body shape is also thought to be a factor in heart disease. Weight concentrated around the abdomen and upper body (making a person apple-shaped) poses a higher health risk than does fat around the hips and thighs of a pear-shaped person.

Lower body fat is almost inert in response to energy needs, and is the last fat to be lost during weight loss diets. Most people lose weight from the top down: face, neck, arms, chest, waist, hips, and, finally, thighs.[2]

Weight-cycling, or yo-yo dieting—losing weight and then gaining it back many times—may have more to do with heart disease than with weight. In one study, 11,000 men who maintained fairly stable body weight between 1962 to 1988 had significantly less heart disease and cardiovascular disease than those men whose weight fluctuated several times over the years. Those who had lost and gained the most pounds had an 80 percent higher rate of heart disease and a 123 percent higher rate of type II diabetes.[3]

Another study, conducted at Stanford University in 1991 found that, among 133 men and 130 women between the ages of 29 and 49, there was a correlation between thigh circumference and heart disease risk: The *larger* the thigh circumference, the *lower* the heart disease risks. A relatively large thigh circumference, especially in women, was associated with both healthful low levels of blood triglycerides and LDL cholesterol (the bad kind), and with high levels of HDL cholesterol (the good kind).[4]

High Blood Pressure and Stress

Obesity is a major risk factor for hypertension. Obesity may cause high blood pressure over time by altering the kidney's physical characteristics and function, leading the body to retain, rather than to eliminate, water. Blood pressure then rises as the body tries to restore the balance of its fluids. Even modest weight loss is beneficial for reducing blood pressure and heart failure.[5] Stress is an even greater risk factor for hypertension: Overweight people who also experience an inordinate amount of negative stress are at increased danger for enlargement of the left heart chamber, one of the major causes of heart failure.

WHAT IS INSULIN RESISTANCE?

Normally, food is absorbed into the bloodstream in the form of sugars (such as glucose), fats, and other basic substances. An increase of glucose in the bloodstream signals the pancreas to release a hormone called insulin. Insulin attaches to cells and allows the glucose to enter them by removing it from the bloodstream.

In insulin resistance, the body's cells have a diminished ability to respond to the action of the insulin. The pancreas then secretes more insulin to compensate for the resistance.

Cholesterol Levels

Visceral obesity is a condition in which deep abdominal fat surrounds internal organs, especially the liver. Usually, visceral obesity is associated with high levels of triglyceride and LDL (bad) cholesterol, and low levels of HDL (good) cholesterol.

In 1992, researchers at Laval University in Quebec used computer-assisted tomography (CT) scans to show that generous amounts of thigh fat seem to counteract the effects of visceral obesity on those with apple-shaped body types. (Apple shapes have more visceral fat than pear shapes.) Men with the fattest thighs had the lowest levels of blood triglycerides and highest levels of HDL (good) cholesterol.

Diabetes

Almost 90 percent of adult-onset diabetics are obese. However, relatively few obese people are diabetic. Many of them are insulin resistant, but have not yet developed the disease.

Researchers blame obesity and sedentary living for the dramatic increase in type II diabetes over the past several years. This may be a result of increased insulin resistance which, in turn, may be caused by increased body fat. It is a complex "falling domino" sequence.

When the amount of fat increases so does insulin resistance; and as insulin resistance increases, more fat is stored. If the fat is near the liver, as in visceral fat, the fatty acids go directly to that organ, which will then be impaired. Impaired liver function can result in high levels of insulin in the blood—a condition called hyperinsulinemia—one of the hallmarks of insulin resistance, which in turn is a forerunner of type II diabetes.

Again, the location of fat on the body seems to be more important than the amount. People who are fat and who participate in sports and exercise programs are not getting diabetes as fast as sedentary adults. The reason may be their lifestyle, rather than their weight.

Cancer

Excess weight may pose a strong risk for esophageal cancer, particularly in young nonsmokers. The increased risk may be due to a higher incidence of gastroesophageal reflux disorder (GERD), also know as chronic heartburn, in people who are overweight.

Obese women appear to have a risk factor two to three times higher than that of normal weight women for uterine cancer and gallbladder cancer. Obese men are at a higher risk for colon and prostate cancers.

There are mixed results on the association between obesity and breast cancer. A number of studies have linked obesity to breast cancer in post-menopausal women. However, in 1990 and 1991, researchers at the University of South Florida College of Medicine reported that women with either endometrial cancer or breast cancer had significantly less thigh fat and smaller hip measurements than women without cancer. Again, the fatter the thighs and the bigger the hips, the lower the risk of these two types of cancer.[6]

Muscles and Bones

Obesity places stress on bones and muscles, and overweight people are at higher risk for hernias, lower back pain, degenerative disc disorders, and aggravation of arthritic conditions and knee problems. Fat people who also consider themselves fit, however, do not seem to have an incidence of joint stress problems or lower back pain any higher than that of their thin and fit counterparts. Therefore, lifting weights and doing aerobic exercise, even while heavy, can offset the greater stress extra weight puts on joints, nerves, and muscles.

Gallstones

The incidence of gallstones is higher than usual in obese women and men. The risk for stone formation is also high if a person loses weight too quickly. In people on very low calorie diets, gallstones may be prevented by taking the prescription drug ursodeoxycholic acid (Actigall). It may be the act of losing and regaining weight, rather than the excess weight itself that promotes gallstone formation.

Reproductive and Hormonal Problems

Women who gain weight after age 18 are at higher risk for developing uterine fibroids. Excess body fat can also contribute to infertility in women, and its dangerous effects on pregnancy are multifold. They include high blood pressure, gestational diabetes, urinary tract infections, blood clots, prolonged labor, higher fetal mortality rate, and Caesarian sections. Women who are obese are also at higher risk for neural tube birth defects such as spina bifida in their babies. In men, obesity can contribute to reduced testosterone levels.

Hypoxia

Obesity puts people at risk for hypoxia, a condition in which oxygen is not sufficient to meet the body's needs. Obese people need to work harder to breathe, and tend to have inefficient respiratory muscles and diminished lung capacity. The Pickwickian syndrome, named for an overweight character in a Dickens novel, occurs in severe obesity—when lack of oxygen produces profound and chronic sleepiness and, eventually, heart failure. Leg aches, numb, cold hands and feet can sometimes be the result of poor circulation, itself the result of a sedentary lifestyle accompanied by obesity. However, cold hands and feet can also occur in thin people if they are not active. It is the lifestyle, rather than the weight, which seems to contribute more to the syndrome.

Sleep Apnea and Sleep Disorders

People who are obese and who nap tend to fall asleep faster and sleep longer during the day. At night, however, it takes longer for them to fall asleep, and they sleep less than people of normal weight.

Obesity is particularly associated with sleep apnea, which occurs when the upper throat relaxes and collapses at intervals during sleep, temporarily blocking the passage of air. Some people may not even know they have this condition except for vague symptoms, such as morning headache, fatigue, and irritability. In a vicious cycle, obesity interferes with sleep and sleep problems may actually contribute to obesity. Lack of restful sleep may contribute to overeating by depriving the person of REM (Rapid Eye Movement) sleep. This dreaming phase of sleep is necessary for long-term emotional well-being, and can leave people less likely to exercise and more tired and sedentary. They may eat to fill a nebulous void in their lives, which is really a lack of sufficient deep sleep.

Binge-Eating and Other Eating Disorders

Roughly 30 percent of people who are obese are binge eaters. Bingeing is defined as consuming 3,000 to 15,000 calories in two hours or less, feeling out of control, and having the problem at least twice a week for six months. For example, eating a whole batch of chocolate chip cookies would equal 5,400 calories if there were 36 cookies at 150 calories each. Add a couple of tall glasses of milk, and a person may exceed 6,000 calories. The person eats rapidly and feels unable stop. They may or may not try to throw up. Binge eating almost always begins before the 20th birthday. Some have surmised that it is an attempt to ease feelings of loneliness. The chart below illustrates the approximate age at which binge eaters begin the behavior.

Age	Percent of All Binge Eaters Who Began at that Age
Before age 10	10 percent
11 to 15	33 percent
16 to 20	43 percent
over age 20	14 percent

A person who occasionally overeats is not considered a binge eater. Some experts believe that binge eating carbohydrates causes an increase in natural opiates, which leads to carbohydrate dependence and should, therefore, be treated as an addiction. Dangerous consequences of binge eating include bulimia and anorexia. Bulimia can result because of an uncomfortable feeling after overeating and the perceived need to get rid of the food by throwing it up and/or using laxatives. Anorexia can appear because the person feels out of control around food and refuses to eat to be in control. Both conditions put the patient at risk for serious medical problems.

Others argue that genetic programming causes binge eating. When sweet and fatty foods—perceived by the body as life sustaining—are eaten, the body craves more. As more food is eaten, more is wanted, just as with a drug addiction. No matter how much sweet and fatty food is consumed, it is never enough. The body gets used to the new, higher levels of endorphins and dopamine in the brain. The body then considers high levels the norm, and wants even more in order to release the same amount of endorphins that a small amount of food once triggered. Dopamine is triggered when food is in the mouth, being smelled, tasted, chewed and swallowed. A huge amount of high-density food is required to feel "normal." and eating spirals out of control. The person becomes addicted to eating a type of food called sugary-fats.[7]

This cycle does have certain characteristics in common with other addictions, in that the body begins to crave more and more, is never satisfied, and suffers withdrawal symptoms if sugary-fats are withheld. These symptoms can include headache, feelings of malaise, depression, lethargy, and overwhelming hunger after having eaten a full meal without sugary-fats. The withdrawal from sugary-fats and the substitution of complex carbohydrates can lead a person away from these cravings.

Social and Emotional Problems

A study that followed obese adolescents for seven years found that, compared to thinner peers, overweight men and women completed fewer years of school, were less likely to be married, and had higher rates of poverty. Sick days, health care costs, and short-term disability all rose as obesity increased. In addition to the societal problems associated with obesity, the toll on each individual is reflected in the number of depressed females, devastated teens, and men in denial about their weight. Whenever an expectation, such as having a near perfect body, cannot be realized, the resulting self-loathing and sadness permeates all aspects of an individual's life.

Childhood Obesity

Fat cells multiply naturally during two growth periods: Early childhood and adolescence. Overeating during these periods increases the number of fat cells. Genetics also determines the number and size of fat cells a person has. One study suggests that though the weight of a toddler does not appear to influence the risk for obesity, an overweight 15-year-old is 17 times more likely to be overweight as an adult than an adolescent of normal weight.[8]

After adolescence, fat cells increase in size, and sometimes in number. Adults who gain weight tend to do so because they have larger fat cells; when those cells are full, they split in two. The only way to remove fat cells is by surgical procedures, such as liposuction or lipectomies (see page 66).

Slender adolescents, who have gained only a few fat cells in their teens, can generally be predicted to remain thin as adults. Weight loss becomes much more difficult for adults who were overweight as children—who may have added substantial numbers of fat cells during their earlier growth spurts. Losing weight in adulthood reduces the size, but not the number, of fat cells.[9]

Studies have shown that, if children have one obese parent, they are 40 percent more likely to become obese adults. If both parents are obese, the likelihood doubles to 80 percent. Since 50 percent of Americans are currently obese, the ratio of fat children to thin children is rising.

Crash diets that are low in protein, and the subsequent yo-yo dieting cycle they often trigger, are significant contributors to obesity. Parents should not attempt to put their child on the diet merry-go-round, but instead encourage increased exercise and healthy eating behaviors. Not allowing snacking while watching TV, and limiting the sedentary hours spent on TV and video games will have a more positive effect on childhood fitness than trying to make a child diet. Criticism of a child's weight puts him or her at greater risk for low self-esteem and withdrawal from activity.[10]

Moose's Story

I am 19, 6-feet tall, and super morbidly obese. I have always been fat and morbidly obese for a long time. When I was 13 I weighed as much as 350-plus pounds. When I was 12 and entering 6th grade, I weighed 275 pounds, and by the end of that year 308 pounds.

To make a long story short, at 14 I kinda took a sojourn from conventional schooling and did my own thing. (My mom made me do home schooling through this home-based charter school and I got my diploma this year.) Well depression plus boredom plus agoraphobia made me gain a good 250 to 300 pounds. So I estimate my current weigh at about 550 to 600 pounds.

As far as weight loss, I went to fat camp two years in a row when I was 13 and 14 losing 50 pounds at first. When I got out of fat camp when I was 13 I was a slim 308 pounds, and a size 46- to 48-inch waist. (That didn't last long.)

The next year I went to the same camp and couldn't be weighed on the scale, but I lost a good 70 pounds, because at the end of the 9 weeks I was on the scale in the 320s.

Well, after that I went back to 8th grade and had crappy year. I didn't like it and took a sojourn at home for half of it.

Somehow along the way, between 14 and 15 I became very agora-phobic. I wasn't at first, but it crept up on me. I think it was due to a large weight gain and people saying the police were gonna arrest me for truancy. This may sound amazing, but I may have gained as much as 200-plus pounds in a year when I was 15 (1999).

When I was 15 I put on a ton of weight, so much that I could bare-ly walk. I was totally inactive, not even going outside to cut the grass. I think I may have weighed 600-plus pounds.

I lost weight from there on my own. It started accidentally when my mom went to Vegas. She had bought food for me for several days while she was gone. I ended up eating it in a few days, so the next few I kinda was hungry. I noticed when my mom got back my shirt was loose. It wasn't skin tight on me. That made me want to start exercising. So, for a few weeks I started doing half sit-ups on my bed, but then stopped a few weeks later. So this was the summer of 1999.

In February 2000, I began to exercise. I started doing 10 sit-ups and five squats. I remember when I first did the sit-ups, it was like the blood hadn't pumped in my heart in years and I was totally exhausted. Well, from that I moved on through the months increasing by five a week until I was doing 500-plus sit-ups and 100-plus squats a day. People don't believe me, but its true. I also was walking during that period. When I first started in February, I went around the block once and was totally exhausted. I just continued, every week increasing by 1 block, until the end of June when I was doing 1 mile a day. I had lost a lot of weight dur-ing those 6 months. I exercised everyday, nonstop, 7 days week. I could almost fit into the pants I was wearing when I started my camp a few years earlier, and I could fit in my mom's seatbelt.

Well, I've gained that all back now since 2000. However I still walk off on and off. I start up again for a month, then don't for 3 or 4, then go 2 months, then stop, and so on, and its been that way since 2000.

I believe that may be the reason I don't have diabetes and am not totally debilitated.

Back in late 1998, Roseanne had a talk show, and by chance I just happened to turn it on one day and she talked about her weight loss. She had Dr. M. Fobi. Well, after that I called for his booklet and have wanted the surgery ever since.

What is the answer for Moose and other young adults like him? If he went on a diet program such as Weight Watchers and lost 1 to 2 pounds a week (as they say you will) it would take him 300 to 400 weeks of consistent dieting to lose the weight. That's six to eight years—if there were no backsliding. How many *adults* can stay on a diet for six weeks, let alone six years?

Moose's genetic makeup favors weight gain and hunger. With either a GBP or a BPD/DS, his hunger signals would diminish, allowing him a chance to relearn how to eat for nutritional benefit. He obviously can be motivated to exercise. With WLS his outlook is hopeful. Without it, it is doubtful he could ever lose the weight on his own.

Our fears and fantasies about our own bodies may be projected onto our children. First is our fear that, if we do not pay constant attention to our bodies, they will get out of control. Second is our fantasy that if we *do* pay attention to them, everything will be fine and we will live beautiful, wonderful lives. Parents may hound or criticize overweight children unfairly because of their own prejudices about being fat. Research indicates that the prejudice of normal weight children against heavy children is worse now than it was in 1961. Children in the 5th and 6th grades were asked to evaluate drawings of six children who were healthy, disabled, or obese. They consistently liked the obese children less—in fact, 40 percent less than in a similar study in 1961.[11]

Children are generally unaware of body types until around ages 5 and 6. In one study, Susan Lewis found that 5 year-olds accurately assessed their own body types only 30 percent of the time (skinny, just right or heavy), while 6-year-olds were accurate 80 percent of the time.[12]

5

How Your Biology Affects Weight-Loss

The cultural bias toward extreme thinness in women has caused an unhealthy and distorted view of what the body should look like. It has created an ideal that is unattainable for most people. Weight loss is difficult enough without a constant barrage of advertising and discrimination (size-ism). Conscious efforts to reduce weight are no match for the biological forces that fight to maintain it.

Obesity and a sedentary lifestyle still pose a threat to life, health, and well-being. A moderate weight loss of 10 or 15 pounds is often beneficial to the quality of life—even if an individual is 50 to 100 pounds overweight—so it is important to understand some of the obstacles that arise when trying to lose weight. We have mistakenly opted to lose fat by reducing our caloric intake, rather than by increasing our expenditure of energy via work or exercise. The body has biological mechanisms in place to prevent this from working. Dieting is one of the reasons that waistlines are expanding.[1]

A number of groups are working to change social perspectives and advocate acceptance of higher weights as a natural.

In 1833, a health formula was proposed by the Morman religious leader, Joseph Smith, who said he was inspired by God. Found in the book, *The Doctrine and Covenants, Section 89,* the doctrine states that whole grains are the basis for nutrition, to be supplemented with herbs, fruits and fresh vegetables in season, and the consumption of very little meat.[2] That formula seems to be accurate, because we find today that a diet rich in complex carbohydrates and fiber, with little animal fat, seems to support good health.

Predictors of Successful Weight Loss

Exercise, problem-solving skills, and social support are the most important predictors of weight loss success. It is not necessarily weight that causes the diseases associated with being overweight; unhealthy foods and a sedentary lifestyle play a large part. In one study, people who began exercising, and who consumed a diet rich in fruits, vegetables and whole grains, experienced significant health gains. After three weeks, indicators for heart disease, blood pressure, and insulin had all improved, although the average weight loss was less than 5 percent.[3] Another study, done in the biosphere in Arizona, found that significant gains in health were accomplished by eating nutritional foods.[4] Other studies have found health gains with only a 5 to 10 percent reduction in weight, as long as the weight stays off. But, with yo-yo dieting, improvements are negligible or even reversed.

Hunger Pangs

Sometimes an obese person cannot rely on hunger pangs as a natural signal to eat. A stomach that has been stretched by large meals or bingeing will often continue to signal hunger until large amounts of food are consumed, or until its size is reduced over time by the consumption of smaller meals. Small meals are considered those that, on average, consist of 1 to 2 cups of food. Quantity eaters sometimes eat 8 to 10 cups of food at one sitting. The non-distended stomach can hold about 4 cups of food diluted with liquid, but less if the food is dry. Therefore, people would feel full more quickly if they avoided drinking liquids with their meals.

Ghrelin, a peptide produced in the stomach, was recently identified. It is a substance that seems to affect the hypothalamus and hunger signals, and has been shown to increase appetite and fat deposits in rats. Injecting ghrelin in higher than normal doses makes rats eat more, and deposit more fat, than a control group. When hybrid rats were bred to produce reduced amounts of ghrelin, the rats were always skinny.[5] This study might hold the key to the future development of anti-hunger pills, if a substance that is able to bind to ghrelin or to render it inactive could be identified.

Low-Fat and High Carbohydrate Diets

Replacing high-fat and sugary foods with low-fat complex carbohydrates may be more effective than calorie counting—particularly for maintaining weight–loss—because dietary fat converts more readily to fat in the body than do carbohydrates or proteins. Therefore, there is a temptation to replace a reduction in fat with an overload of simple carbohydrates. Keep in mind that excess calories from any source will add pounds.

In one study, a group of men were fed a typical American diet of 35 percent fat, plus enough calories per day from other sources to maintain their weight. After a couple of weeks, they were switched to a diet consisting of the same number of calories, but with only 15 percent of these calories coming from fat. The remaining 85 percent of the calories came from unrefined foods. The men maintained their weight, but complained that they could not eat all the food they were given.[6]

Switching to low-fat dairy products may help achieve recommended dietary goals. Fat substitutes that are added to "low-fat" commercial foods, or used in baking, deliver some of the qualities of fat, but do not add as many calories. Some of these substitutes, such as cellulose gel, carrageenan, guar gum, and gum arabic, have been used for decades in commercial foods and are recognized as safe.

Fat and Sugar Substitutes

Olestra, one of the newer synthetic fats, contains fat molecules that are too large to be absorbed by the body. However, people have reported experiencing cramps and diarrhea after eating food containing Olestra, and a small percentage of people seem to be sensitive to it. Olestra also depletes the body of fat-soluble vitamins and disease-fighting nutrients. This decrease may put a person at risk for cancer, stroke, and heart disease. Studies conducted by John Blundell in Leeds, England, demonstrated that people given Olestra in a meal made up for the fewer calories by eating more later in the day. His conclusion: you may be able to fool your taste buds—but not your brain.[7]

Simplesse is another fat substitute currently marketed under the brand name Simple Pleasures. This synthetic fat has a pleasing creamy texture, but cannot be used in cooking because it breaks down when exposed to high heat. Other fat-substitutes, derived from oats (Oat Trim and Z-Trim), are currently being investigated.

Fiber—such as the pectin found in apples and other fruits—has also been associated with prolonging feelings of fullness after eating.

Sugar substitutes like saccharin, aspartame (NutraSweet, Equal), acesulfame K (Sweet One) and sucralose (Splenda) are good alternatives to sugar for those attempting to lose weight. Acesulfame and sucralose usually leave no bitter aftertaste in baking, as do saccharin and aspartame. The bitter aftertaste is caused when ingredients in the artificial sugars bind with the bitter taste sensors in the mouth.

Early studies found that large amounts of saccharin caused cancer in rats, but such large quantities would be unpalatable to humans.

Aspartame has come under scrutiny because of rare reports of neurological disorders, including headaches or dizziness. However, an association with brain cancer is unfounded. Some people are sensitive to one compound, and some to another. Sugar substitutes are generally safe for consumption if one uses common sense.

Extreme Diets

Any diet that advocates the consumption of fewer than 1,500 calories a day carries health risks and is often followed by episodes of bingeing or overeating and a return to obesity. Severe weight loss has also been linked to fatigue, intolerance to cold, hair-loss, gallstones, and menstrual irregularities.

Most initial weight loss consists of fluid and minerals; fat is lost later on, along with muscle. Muscle loss can account for 30 percent of the weight lost. Because of the risk of muscle and nutrient loss, it is dangerous to remain on an extreme diet for more than 16 weeks.

High-Protein / High-Fat Diets

High-protein diets, such as the Atkins diet, lead to quick weight loss, but the health benefits are dubious. Ketones—substances produced when the body breaks down fats for energy—are among the by-products associated with these diets and can cause nausea, lightheadedness and bad breath. A ketone diet can be an effective weight loss regimen for morbidly obese patients only if they are carefully monitored by health professionals through-out the diet. However, there is a reported increase in the propensity to gain the weight back, and then some, when such a diet is stopped. Dr. Atkins himself admitted this shortcoming in an interview on the television program *Oprah,* in May 2000.

Frequent, Short Periods of Exercise

Frequent exercise sessions as short as 10 minutes may be most effective for the obese individuals. This is partly because it is eas-ier to find time and motivation for a 10-minute session than for one that lasts for 30 to 45 minutes. Although brief workouts do not burn great numbers of calories, metabolism will remain ele-vated for a time after exercise. So, even if only a few calories have been lost, over time they will contribute significantly to main-taining a healthy weight. The more strenuous the exercise, the longer the metabolism will continue to burn calories before returning to its resting level.

Exercise also improves psychological well-being and replaces the sedentary habits that lead to snacking. Exercise even acts as an appetite suppressant. Other small changes, such as using the stairs, parking a distance away from a destination, taking a longer route instead of a short-cut, and never eating in the car can enhance the effects of saving or consuming modest amounts of calories. Eventually, these small habits make a difference. A 21-pound weight gain over a 5-year period represents only a fraction—1.5 percent—of the 4 to 5 million calories consumed and used as energy during that period. Those excess calories could have been burned as energy by additional walking or stair climbing. By eating only one or two bites less at each meal, a person could meet the goal of eating 1.5 percent fewer calories per day, and weight-gain would not be a problem.

The difference in calorie consumption between an average weight individual and a super obese person (see Chapter 9) is around 250 calories per day—or two cups of milk.[8]

An exercise regimen consisting of short bursts of energy of 10 minutes each, at least 15 times each week, along with an increase in the amount of fiber in the diet, is advocated in the book, *The Spark*.[9] Authors Glenn Gaessar, MD, and Karla Dougherty measured parameters such as metabolic fitness, muscle endurance, flexibility, body fat, cholesterol, triglycerides, sleep, and muscle and joint aches. All parameters were improved after just three weeks on their Spark program. According to Gaesser:

As we age and put on weight, we lose our ability to produce and secrete growth hormone (GH), which, in our youth, made our bones strong, our bodies supple, our immune system hearty. GH can seemingly turn back the clock. GH injections are available, but only to the rich. . . . With the right kind of activity, three times a day, your own body is stimulated once again to release this hormone, naturally, safely. . . . Your body is continually producing and secreting GH when you exercise for short bouts (Spark program) a few times a day. But, when you exercise only once a day, your body compensates, slowing down the GH secretions—regardless of how long that session may be. In the same way your metabolism shuts down when you starve yourself on a stringent diet, GH goes into slow motion. Your body feels the need to conserve its valuable surge of GH and, as the day goes on, you get less and less output. In other words, you might think you're turning back the clock when you push yourself through a 45-minute Tae-Bo class, but, in reality, you're going to be secreting less and less GH throughout the day. . . . If you're spending 45 minutes in the gym and that's it for the day, your body compensates later—by producing and secreting less GH! If you only did a couple of easy kick-boxing moves throughout the day (10-minute kicks, three times a day!), you'd actually keep yourself younger—longer.[10]

Other Factors

Doctors have known for decades about thyroxin and adrenaline, two body chemicals that increase metabolism. When thyroxin is given in high enough doses, it speeds weight loss. However, it also causes thyrotoxicosis—anxiety, fast heart rate, heart palpitations, protruding eyes, sleeplessness, sweating, and tremors. The other chemical is adrenaline, which directs your fight-or-flight response, and causes alertness, sweating, goose bumps and dilation of the pupils. Unfortunately, the negatives outnumber the positives. Side effects are just too uncomfortable to bear, even if the chemicals are able to burn fat.

Even when stomach surgery is not tied to weight loss—such as surgery due to stomach cancer—doctors still find it results in a profound lack of appetite. "These patients aren't hungry. You would expect they would be really hungry. This is the most intriguing aspect of bariatric surgery. If we can understand what makes people hungry and what takes hunger away in people who have gastric surgery, maybe we can find a nonsurgical solution to obesity."[11]

Obesity may not be a direct cause of disease, but it and many other diseases serve as *markers* for an imprudent lifestyle. Excessive consumption of alcohol, fat, and sugar, and inadequate exercise and dietary fiber all contribute to disease, and can certainly result in weight-gain. If these lifestyle factors are the true culprits in obesity-related disease, the current focus on weight-reduction may be misplaced, and healthy nutrition with increased activity a preferable alternative. Even though obesity is overwhelmingly genetic, environmental factors are important, too. If a village of Nepalese citizens were transported to America, it is probable that within a few years they would begin to experience the same weight problems that Americans do, even though there are very few overweight individuals in Nepal. It is the advertisement and consumption of processed foods and sedentary lifestyles that make us fat.

Why We Give Up On Diets

After beginning a diet, many people become discouraged because weight loss slows. This phenomenon is widespread. After the first couple of weeks on any weight loss program, you have to exercise more in order to maintain weight loss.

Unfortunately, the reverse usually happens. Surveys by the Centers for Disease Control and Prevention (CDC) indicate that 25 percent of adults are completely sedentary—that is, they get no exercise at all and 54 percent are not active enough to reap any health benefits. Guidelines from the NIH define 30 minutes of exercise three times a week as "moderately active." Newer research shows that shorter, multiple periods of exercise every day provide even greater benefits.

6

Diet Drugs

Over-the-Counter (OTC) Drugs and Herbal Remedies

Caution should be used with over-the-counter herbal remedies. For instance, the *herbal* weight loss medication phen-fen (Herbal Phen-Fen, PhenTrim, Phen-Cal) contains ephedrine, which is derived from the ephedra (also known as Ma Huang). Some people may experience severe side effects, such as rapid heartbeat, high blood pressure, psychosis, and seizures after ingesting small amounts of ephedrine.

Dietary teas and supplements that list plantain as an ingredient contain digitalis, a powerful chemical that affects the heart. Many teas contain laxatives and can cause gastrointestinal distress and, if overused, lead to chronic pain, constipation, and dependency. Some laxative substances found in teas include senna, aloe, buckthorn, rhubarb root, cascara (which is very powerful) and castor oil.

Following are some herbal remedies that have a high potential for helping in weight management. As with any medication, some may work for one person but not for another. Some are thermogenic, which means that they boost metabolism; others help control appetite.

Carnitine (L-Carnitine)

Carnitine, a nonessential amino acid, has a thermogenic affect. Studies suggest that it helps overcome the effects that high cholesterol and lipids have on the immune system in people who are obese. Side effects are nausea and diarrhea.[1]

Cayenne (Capsacin)

As a thermogenic agent that promotes blood flow and perspiration, cayenne can increase metabolism by 2.5 percent when 1 teaspoon red pepper sauce and 1 teaspoon mustard are taken with meals. It should be taken with food to protect the stomach. Hot sensations in the mouth or the anus during a bowel movement are primary side effects. Cayenne does not seem to cause ulcers; in fact, it improves digestion and relieves gas.

Citrus Aurantium (zhi shi)

Zhi shi is a thermogenic agent derived from the rind of the bitter orange. It has been used in Chinese medicine to treat indigestion and to promote circulation and liver health. A scientific study in 1999[2] examined the anti-obesity effects in rats, and found that citrus aurantium significantly reduced food intake and weight-gain. It has no known side effects, and does not increase heart rate or blood pressure.

Coenzyme Q10 (ubiquinone)

Coenzyme Q10, a thermogenic agent, is a naturally occurring antioxidant found in cells throughout the body. Levels decline as people age, and many believe that supplementation may slow down the aging process. Although there are studies focusing on its capacity for reducing the risk of heart attack and for lowering blood pressure, little research has been done on it as a weight loss agent. However, an exploratory study found that individuals with a family history of obesity had both a 50 percent-reduced ability to burn calories after eating, *and* low CoQ10 levels.[3] There are no known side effects.

Conjugated Linoleic Acid (CLA)

CLA is a thermogenic agent found naturally in dairy products, beef, poultry, and corn oil. Animal studies have shown a loss in fat mass when taking CLA. One of the few human studies shows that volunteers given CLA for 3 months lost 20 percent of their body fat, and increased lean muscle mass.[4] Side effects may include gastrointestinal disturbance.

Dehydroepiandrosterone (DHEA)

A thermogenic agent, DHEA is a weak androgen, or male hormone, that is present in both sexes. Its levels rapidly decline as we age. Much research has been done on the anti-aging properties of DHEA, but not on its effects on weight loss. Some claim that DHEA promotes fat burning by preventing the action of an enzyme necessary for fat production. Side effects may include acne, fatigue, insomnia, irritability, breast enlargement in some men, and facial hair and deepening of the voice in women. It can also cause heart palpitations in some people. Long-term effects may include an increase in tumors and cancer.

5-hydroxytryptophan (5-HTP)

The amino acid 5-HTP is a chemical precursor of the neurotransmitter serotonin, which modulates mood, emotion, sleep, and appetite. 5-HTP is naturally produced in the body. It is hypothesized that people who have a decreased ability to convert tryptophan to 5-HTP (and thus have low levels of serotonin) are more likely to be obese and to suffer from depression. In animal studies, rats that were bred to overeat and that were fed 5-HTP ate less than expected.[5] Human studies seem to show that taking 5-HTP helps in reducing carbohydrate intake. Side effects include a bloated feeling, flatulence, heartburn, and nausea.

Glucomannan

Extracted from the konnyaku root—a member of the yam family—glucomannan is also known as devil's tongue and voodoo lily. This water-soluble dietary fiber is a good source of beta-carotene, thiamin, and minerals. Human experiments have been flawed, but seem to indicate that people who take glucomannan can lose as much as a pound a week and lower their cholesterol levels without changing their eating habits.

Glucomannan reduces the body's ability to absorb vitamin E and other nutrients; its consumption should be monitored by a physician.

Guar Gum (Cyamopsis Tetragonoloa)

Guar gum is a complex carbohydrate used as a laxative. When it comes in contact with liquids, it forms a heavy, viscous mass, causing people to feel full. It also hinders fat absorption.

In 1992, guar gum was banned from use in diet products after some people experienced a blockage of their gastrointestinal tract after using the product incorrectly. It was later found that these people had failed to drink enough liquid when they took guar gum. With the passage of the 1994 Dietary Supplement Health and Education Act, guar gum was recognized as generally safe when used correctly. It produces no side effects if taken with a full glass of water and used as directed. Guar gum is found in most ice creams and many other food products.

Guggul (Commiphora Mukul)

As a thermogenic agent, guggul has been used for weight management in ayurvedic medicine for 2,000 years. It may increase the secretion of thyroid hormone and stimulate the body to burn calories more efficiently. However, for people with heart disease, guggul can cause unwanted stimulatory effects.

Over-the-Counter Human Growth Hormone Enhancers (Liddel Vital HGH, Physician's Choice Super HGH)

These OTC enhancers—not to be confused with costly GH available by injection—stimulate the body's production of growth hormone (GH). The various enhancers on the market contain substances that affect the actions of growth hormone and somatostatin. There are studies that show a decrease in body fat after several weeks on the enhancer. Side effects may include mild joint pain during the initial course of medication. It may also cause insulin resistance and can aggravate diabetes.

Maitake (Grifola frondosa)

Maitake is a mushroom that promotes weight loss. Animal and human studies seem to support this claim. It has no known side effects. It can be found in most Asian food stores as a dried mushroom.

Psyllium

Psyllium plays a role in reducing cholesterol and fat levels in the blood. Because the mucilage in psyllium husks absorbs fluid, it creates a feeling of fullness when it makes contact with water after eating. Psyllium may cause abdominal cramps, bloating, and flatulence in some people.

Prescription Diet Drugs

Drugs prescribed for weight loss are generally called anorexiants, because they suppress hunger. Most lose their effectiveness over time and require increasing dosages, and many can become addictive.

When you take diet drugs, you lose weight; but when you stop taking them you will gain the weight back. Drugs do not *cure* obesity—they can only help control it.

There are many contraindications to the use of diet drugs. They include alcoholism, anorexia, concurrent use of migraine medication, drug abuse, hypertension, lactation, pregnancy, psychosis, and use of MAO inhibitors or lithium. Other relative contraindicators are depression or concurrent use of SSRI antidepressants, glaucoma, and heart, kidney or liver abnormalities. These latter conditions need to be evaluated by a physician before diet drugs are prescribed.

Benzphetamine (Didrex)

Approved by the FDA in 1960, benzphetamine is an appetite suppressant with moderate potential for abuse. It works by stimulating satiety (fullness) in the hypothalamus and limbic regions of the brain. Side effects include nervousness, irritability, headache, sweating, dry mouth, nausea, insomnia and constipation.

Diethylpropion hydrochloride (Depletite, Tenuate, Tepanil, and generic)

Diethylpropion hydrochloride is an appetite suppressant that increases blood pressure, slows the heart, and stimulates the central nervous system. It was approved in 1959, and is a schedule IV drug, with low potential for abuse.

At the end of a placebo controlled double-blind study, those on the drug had lost an average of 15.9 pounds compared to those in the control group, who had lost 10 pounds. Side effects include insomnia and irritability.[6]

Fluoxetine (Prozac)

Prozac is an antidepressant that is sometimes prescribed as an anorexiant (appetite suppressant). Side effects may include fatigue, diarrhea, sweating, headache, insomnia, vomiting, nausea, thirst, and impaired sexual function.

Mazindol (Mazinor, Sanorex)

Mazindol, a schedule IV controlled substance with a low potential for abuse, is a nonamphetamine appetite suppressant. It reduces appetite by directly blocking the feeding control center, located in the hypothalamus.

Approved in 1973, Mazindol is the only anti-obesity drug licensed in Japan. In 1996, Japanese researchers tested the drug on dieters coming off a low-calorie diet. They found that the women lost an additional 15 pounds after three months of treatment with the drug, without the diet. The women in the control group began to regain lost weight. Mazindol or a placebo was also given to 228 obese patients for 12 weeks. The treated patients had more significant appetite and weight reduction than placebo-treated patients, an average of 18 pounds at a dosage of 3 milligrams per day.[7] Side effects can include nervousness, restlessness, insomnia, euphoria, and overstimulation.

Orlistat (Xenical)

Orlistat is an inhibitor of gastrointestinal lipases; it blocks 30 percent of dietary fat from being absorbed. In studies of people taking Orlistat, cholesterol levels improved more than expected because of its direct inhibition of fat absorption. Orlistat administration to an at-risk population over a four-year period reduced the progression to type II diabetes more effectively than diet and exercise alone.

Patients put on Orlistat alone achieved a 10-percent weight loss in one year. During the second year, patients who continued on the drug gained back only half as much weight as patients who were given a placebo. Multivitamin supplementation is recommended for this regimen because Orlistat can reduce the absorption of lipid-soluble vitamins. Side effects can be significant, and include uncontrolled gas, liquid bowel movements, and gastrointestinal pain.

Some people taking the drug report that they pass what they think is gas, only to find that they have, in fact, discharged a brown or yellow liquid. This oily liquid soaks readily through fabric and is hard to remove by laundering. This side effect can present serious social consequences.

Phentermine (Adipex-P, Dapex, Fastin, Ioniman, Obe-Nix, Obephen, Obermine, Obestin-30, Ona-Mast, Parmine, Phetrol, T-Diet, Termine, Unifast Unicelles, and Wilpowr)

Phentermine is an appetite suppressant and central nervous system stimulant, formerly part of the combination product Phentermine Fenfluramine (Phen-Fen or Fen-Phen). Approved for weight management in 1973, it is a schedule IV controlled substance with low potential for abuse.

Phentermine stimulates the feeding center in the hypothalamus and limbic regions of the brain, where appetite and hunger are controlled. To be effective it must be used in conjunction with a sensible eating plan and exercise. Weight loss is only temporary, and the dosage needs to be increased to continue the results. Side effects include dry mouth, nausea, sleeplessness, headache, stomach upset, constipation, and irritability.

Phendimetrazine (Adipost, Adphen, Anorex, Bacarat, Bontrilm Dyrexan-OD, Metra, Obalan, Phnzine, Statobex, Trimstat, and Wehless)

An appetite suppressant and amphetamine-like stimulant, Phendimetrazine is a schedule III controlled substance with a moderate potential for abuse. Weight loss may be temporary, and side effects included restlessness, insomnia, dizziness, tremors, heart palpitations, blurred vision, constipation, dry mouth and change in sex drive.

Sibutrimine (Meridia)

Sibutramine balances serotonin, norepinephrine, and dopamine (all neurotransmitters), and increases metabolism. People show significant weight loss and reduction in risk factors relating to diabetes. It was developed in the late 1980s as an anti-depressant and, in 1997, as a weight loss aid.

Sibutrimine causes a feeling of fullness and increases energy levels. Side effects can include dry mouth and insomnia. Some have reported high blood pressure and abnormal heart rhythms. Many conditions prohibit the use of sibutramine in conjunction with other drugs. Long-term effects have not been studied on patients who are taking this drug, so whether weight loss can be maintained is still questionable.

Amphetamines (Addererall, Biphetamine)

Amphetamines have a high potential for abuse and are less effective than many other medications in helping to maintain weight loss. Amphetamines elevate mood and produce modest weight loss over the short term, but also present serious risks of addiction, agitation, and insomnia. Additionally, when a person regains normal hunger signals, they tend to overeat because of the deprivation they felt while on the drugs. Amphetamine-like drug include Ritalin and Concerta.

Experimental Therapies

Amylin is a peptide that can slow the emptying of the stomach. When Amylin and CCK (see below) are used in combination, each enhances the effect of the other. However, in order to be potent, it must be injected. Experiments with a nasal spray are being tested.

Choecystokinin (CCK) is released into the bloodstream and increases the feeling of fullness when food (especially fat and protein) reaches the small intestine. The body's normal release of CCK is triggered by distention of the stomach, which activates nerve messages that travel to the hypothalamus.

Several companies are trying to develop a CCK-like drug. The problem is that CCK is a peptide (a small protein) and, when taken orally, it is broken down and deactivated by digestive enzymes in the mouth. The Fisons pharmaceutical company has had some success in animal studies with CCK administered by intranasal spray. The strategy employed by Eli Lilly, Glaxo, and Hoffman La Roche is to create a peptoid, which is smaller than a peptide. To date, the CCK peptoids that retain activity cannot be absorbed, and the ones that *can* be absorbed have lost biologic activity.

Enterostatin, which is made in the pancreas, blocks the desire to eat fat. Several animal studies have demonstrated the ability of the man-made drug to prevent fat intake without effects on car-bohydrates or proteins. It can be given by mouth, or injected, and trials are under way.

Growth Hormone Treatment. A combination treatment of growth hormone and an insulin-like substance was shown to improve fat-loss when added to diet and exercise in post-menopausal obese women. The drug is administered by self-injection, and can cause water retention and swelling. Unfortunately, the present cost is prohibitively expensive for most people.

Leptin is a substance that occurs naturally in the body, and has a role in regulating hunger. It is supposed to be a sweet-sensing modulator (suppressor) that may take part in regulating food intake. Doubling the concentration of leptin in the blood of mice suggested that it might prove to be an effective drug in the treatment of obesity. However in humans, there is only a .01 percent chance that obesity occurs because of leptin insufficiency.

Preliminary results from early studies reported that patients taking the highest dose of this drug lost 8 percent of their body weight after 6 months, and indicated that the drug was well tolerated. Leptin affects the sense of taste, suppressing responses of peripheral taste nerves to sweet substances without affecting their responses to sour, salty and bitter. Tests on humans are contradictory, but most report that the drug does not live up to its promise.

Naltrexone. This drug, sold under the name *Trexan,* blocks the euphoria of drug abusers, and is being tested on people who binge eat as a preventative. (Binge eating is defined as consuming 3,000 to 15,000 calories in less than two hours, at least twice a week, for six months.) Trexan's effects have been promising. It has no effect on non-bingers and is only available by injection.

Neuropeptide Y (NPY), Galanin, and Ghrelin. These are peptides, found naturally in the body, that strongly stimulate food intake. If a product could be developed that effectively *blocked* these peptides, a new tool in the fight against obesity would be available.

Photo Therapy. Bright light has an effect on melatonin, a powerful hormone that regulates sleep and other functions, and also positively affects serotonin levels. It is beneficial for depression caused by the shorter days and reduced light of seasonal changes (Seasonal Affective Disorder, or SAD).

Lux is the international unit of illumination. One small study, in which participants were exposed to 1,500 lux each morning for 30 minutes, reported that three out of four women who were sensitive to the effects of light lost between three and five pounds after 10 days.[8]

Rimonabant (Acomplia). A new pill in the final stages of testing shows promise in attacking both smoking and hunger levels. It seems to shut down addictive oral cravings. The French developer, Sanofi-Synthelabo, plans to seek approval to sell it in the U.S. in 2005.[9]

Topiramate (Topamax). Currently used as an anti-seizure medication and a treatment for migraine headaches, Topiramate has an unexpected side effect and off-label use as a weight loss drug. A two-week titration to an appropriate dosage is recommended. Side effects of dry mouth seem to be well tolerated, and the drug seems to work effectively on sweet tooth cravings. Topiramate is currently undergoing clinical trials to approve its use for weight-control. Side effects of headache and nausea can occur when patients are withdrawn from this drug abruptly, and should be monitored by a doctor.[10]

Weight-Loss Attempts

Although there has been, and continues to be, research in the area of weight loss, so far nothing seems to work for the long term; 97 percent of the people who try any one or more of the above products regain the weight lost. Only 3 percent are able to change environmental and behavior factors enough so that permanent weight loss can be maintained. Neurotransmitters carry messages from the brain with chemical messengers including serotonin and dopamine. One of the reasons that people like to eat is that both serotonin and dopamine (powerful feel-good chemicals) are stimulated by the act of chewing, tasting, smelling, and swallowing food. Serotonin activity also increases markedly in response to the consumption of carbohydrates.[11] Group support programs such as Weight Watchers, TOPS, and Jenny Craig flourish because of excellent short-term results. However, such programs seldom succeed in the maintenance of desired weight loss, leading to many more attempts with the same program before a person gives up. Some people return to the same programs 25 to 50 times during their lifetimes because of their proven initial success, not realizing that the same program has led to just as many failures. They blame themselves, not the program.

Weight loss continues to be big business. In the United States, as many as one-third of women surveyed are on a diet at any one time. The proof of dismal success rates does not seem to deter continued efforts to lose weight. New diets and pills are quickly replaced with others, and the battle goes on.

The only weight loss method for morbidly obese people that has a high percentage of positive long-term results is weight loss surgery. Significant weight loss occurs in at least 80 percent of patients followed for five years and longer. However, severe side effects make this a last resort for the truly obese.

7

How Dieting Leads to Weight Gain

Many people go on diets again and again, even though they are never successful in the long run. What is motivation to go on yet another diet? The following diary is a possible scenario that explains to some extent why diets are so attractive, at least at first, when the weight comes off quickly and the body has not gone into starvation mode.

Diary of a Diet

Preliminary thoughts:

1. I've got to do something about my weight.
2. I'm gaining weight. I've gained 10 pounds in the last two months.
3. I'll try eating less and exercising more.
4. Wait a minute, I'm still gaining. I *know* I don't eat that much.
5. Why am I so hungry all the time?

6. What method has worked in the past? Weight Watchers, Jenny Craig, (or any other diet programs) have worked. I'm going to rejoin.
7. Before I start, I better eat all the stuff around the house I know I can't have when I'm being serious.

On the Diet

1. This is great. I know this will work, I've done it before.
2. This isn't so hard; I can have all this food to eat.
3. I really like eating this way, I feel so healthy.
4. I can plan what I want to eat in advance.
5. Why didn't I start this sooner?

A Week or Two Later

1. I'm *so* hungry—and I've already eaten all the food I'm allowed today.
2. Why did I eat a fast food burger? That's half my food for the day.
3. Why did I eat those Girl Scout cookies? I could've had just two, but I ate the whole box.
4. It's so hard to plan what I'm going to eat in advance because I'm always so hungry.
5. There were muffins at work and I had two. Oh no, I can't eat dinner now.
6. I've been so good, but I've stopped losing.
7. It must be my menstrual cycle—I'm so hungry.
8. I can't eat like this forever.
9. I want to eat whatever I want.
10. I've lost a few pounds. It's okay now, the crisis is over.

11. I'm so much happier when I eat what I want. I'll just eat less and exercise more.

Later Still

1. Why did I go off that diet? I could be ten pounds lighter now if I had just stayed on it.
2. I keep gaining weight.
3. This is the heaviest I've ever been.
4. I've got to do something.
5. What has worked before? I think I'll rejoin.

Studies of Yo-Yo Dieting

According to Maarit Korkeila, a nutritionist at the University of Helsinki, weight loss attempts appear to increase the risk of long-term major weight gain in adults. She says that the relationship between weight loss attempts and weight gain can be partially attributed to a familial predisposition to gain weight. She and fellow researchers followed more than 7,500 men and women, ages 18 to 54, for 15 years. They recorded weight, dieting, and other factors such as educational level, alcohol use, social class, and marital status. Results showed that nearly all the normal weight subjects who attempted to diet gained more than 10 pounds over the next 15 years. The success rate of dieting was approximately 3 percent, with the other 97 percent failing not only to maintain their weight, but also actually gaining a substantial amount of weight. Those who did not attempt to diet stayed within 3 percent of their original weight 15 years later.[1] This large sample is the most comprehensive study of dieting and weight-gain attempted to date.

The first evidence of the negative effects of dieting was discovered in a landmark study conducted by Dr. Ancel Keys in 1944.[2] Thirty-two conscientious objectors had been assigned to alternative service during World War II, and were living in university dormitories. In Dr. Keys' study, the subjects lived on a diet made up of slightly less than half the calories they were accustomed to for 24 weeks. As expected, all the men lost weight. And, also as expected, they all put the weight back on when they were allowed to go off the diet. But they did not regain just the weight they had lost; most gained several pounds *more* than that, all in the form of fat. Six of the men gained an average of 9 1/2 pounds more body fat than they'd had before entering what became, in effect, the first controlled experiment in "yo-yo" dieting.[3]

Identical twins are often studied to identify the effect of genetics on a particular trait. In one study at St. Vincent's Hospital in Australia, twins were given a lengthy questionnaire about physical activities and diet. The study compared their answers, and at least one of each pair considered themselves to be overweight. If genetics are so powerful, could one twin be heavy and the other of normal weight? The twin who consistently exercised at a moderate pace carried, on average, 6 pounds less body fat than the inactive twin. Vigorous exercisers had 12 fewer pounds of fat. This study confirms the fact that a genetic tendency to be overweight can be offset by daily exercise.

However, within the three body types, ectomorph (naturally thin), mesomorph (normal weight), and endomorph (overweight), each set of twins as a unit was characterized by one of the three categories. The difference in their weights, from one twin to the other, were slight, and varied only from six to 25 pounds. In one case, both twins were mesomorphs; one weighed 145 pounds and the other, who exercised less, weighed 157 pounds. In another case, both twins were endomorphs, with one twin weighing 200 pounds and the other, 225 pounds. In only 5 percent of the cases were these identical twins of different body types.

A study of 1,700 sets of twins who had different environmental histories concluded that, over the long-term, dieters are doomed to failure. The main culprit in weight gain is believed to be the makeup of the individual, with a predisposition to gain weight based on genetics, rather than on environment. In that study, researchers followed 3,400 identical twins who were raised apart from one another. When one twin had a weight problem and attempted to diet, the other twin invariably had a similar weight problem, with or without dieting. Their adult weights seemed to be predetermined, and were not a function of family eating patterns or dieting failures. Both members of the identical twins groups were within a few pounds of each other, whether or not they had dieted. If one was thin, the other had a 95 percent chance of being thin. If one was obese, the other also had a 95 percent chance of being obese, despite dieting attempts by either one of the twins.[4]

Feeling Full

Feeling full after a meal is the result of at least two signals to stop eating that are generated by the stomach and the small intestine. When food and drink distend the stomach, they activate nerve messages that travel to the hypothalamus. When food (especially fat and protein) reaches the small intestine, CCK is released into the bloodstream and increases the feeling of fullness.

Some patients seem to have a faulty hormone release mechanism, and thus do not feel full after eating a normal amount of food. These patients constantly overeat because they do not feel full until after they have eaten 8 to 10 cups or more of food, and have caused their stomachs to swell considerably. It is not known whether this behavior is learned, or whether it is genetically determined.

People often hear the term "shrink your stomach." The stomach does not shrink, but it *can* expand. For example, a person's stomach may hold only 4 cups of food. However, a person who chronically eats 8 cups of food will stretch his or her stomach to hold that much; thus he or she gets used to feeling full only after 8 cups of food have been eaten.

When that person goes on a diet and eats less food, the stomach returns to its original size of 4 cups. The stomach seems to have shrunk, but in fact has simply returned to its original size.

An initial criticism of gastric bypass was that obese people would not be able to give up eating huge amounts of food. Research indicates levels of ghrelin—a hunger inducing enzyme—spike before meals, and are at their lowest during the night. It has also been reported that bypass patients secrete almost no ghrelin, and so do not crave large quantities of food (See page 73 for more information about ghrelin). Restrictive procedures, such as the adjustable gastric band surgery (see page 16), do not cause a reduction in hunger signals, because all of the stomach remains active.[5]

8

The Problem with Diets

The biggest problem with diets usually confronts us only after the diet is over. The weight lost almost never *stays* off because our bodies naturally have what is known as a *set-point*, determined by our genes and basic body type. (See Body Types on page 32.)

This set-point is not necessarily the point at which our weight naturally stays if we do everything right—though that may very well be the set-point of a thin person (ectomorph). The set-point for a fat person (endomorph) seems to be their last heaviest weight, until they finally reach the weight pre-determined by their genes and body type.

The body works hard to get us to our set-point by increasing hunger and the rate at which we absorb food and calories in our intestines. The body can also go into *starvation mode*, holding onto every single calorie and fat particle it can until we reach our set-point.

Many women who gain a moderate amount of weight during pregnancy notice that, after giving birth, they return to their last heaviest weight. It does not matter that they were pregnant at the time. Their bodies do not seem to make the distinction. Pregnancy is one time during adulthood when fat cells increase in number as a natural phenomenon. During subsequent pregnancies, the cycle repeats until, depending on how many children a woman has had, she becomes morbidly obese. This is one of the reasons more women are obese than men. Another reason women tend to be heavier is that more men have jobs that involved physical labor, while women's jobs tend to be more sedentary.

Dieting is an attempt to thwart the set-point; the winner in the eating contest is not willpower, but biologically driven urges to consume ever greater amounts of food (to reach our natural set-point). The big winner is the weight loss industry. Our bodies have given the industry the perfect strategy to keep us stuck in a vicious cycle of weight loss and weight-gain. We are told that the dieter failed, not the diet. When Oprah Winfrey lost 67 pounds on the Optifast (liquid diet) program, sales for the company soared. When she regained the weight, she hired a chef and a personal trainer and, with a great deal of effort, was able to maintain a reasonable weight for a while.

Oprah Winfrey and her personal trainer, Bob Greene, co-authored the book, *Make the Connection,* which offers excellent advice about making lifestyle changes to become fit. However, since she is genetically programmed to be overweight, only a vigilant preoccupation with food and exercise keeps her thin. The alternative—to be beautifully dressed, coiffed, happy and fit, but not pencil thin—seems to be the path she has chosen at present, and she is a great role-model for who cannot seem to win the battle of the bulge.

Loss of Lean Muscle Mass

Another contributor to obesity is the loss of lean muscle mass that happens naturally as we age. A long illness, time in bed, crash diets, and lack of exercise can all contribute to decreasing metabolism because of a decrease in muscle. Muscle proteins start to undergo change in as little as 24 hours of inactivity. Since muscles use energy, more muscle mass equals more energy expenditure. That is why weight-bearing exercise and weight lifting increase overall muscle mass, and non-weight bearing exercises, such as swimming, are less effective.

Super Absorbers

Fat people tend to be super-absorbers. The old notion that calories in plus energy expended equals weight gain or loss is not exactly true for everyone. Some people can eat 5,000 calories a day and not gain weight; others gain weight on fewer than 2,000 calories a day. Male prison inmates volunteered to eat huge amounts of food each day to see how much weight they could gain over six months, but were permitted to exercise as much as they wanted. Each participant had maintained a stable weight for at least one year prior to the study. Though all the inmates were eating the same high-calorie diet, some of them gained 20 pounds, others gained 40 pounds, and some gained nothing at all. Because exercise levels were not monitored, we can assume the men who gained no weight probably increased their exercise levels. It is also probable that the lucky men who gained little or no weight were somehow able to convert excess calories by dissipating them internally through thermogenics (heat).

Thermogenics is simply a faster metabolism. It determines the body's ability to utilize energy in the form of glycogen or fat, to give off heat, and thus to burn calories. This can be accomplished through movement, digestion, brain activity, sweating, shivering, and the operation and maintenance of all bodily functions. Those people who have an ability to burn more calories seem to have a built in control that expends heat through fidgeting, movement during sleep, excess sweating, faster digestion, as well as hormonal and endocrine system signals that drive a person to exercise and to be more active.

A similar study reported the same effect. Two dozen subjects were overfed by 1,000 calories per day. The study supervisors did not want the subjects to exercise, or try to compensate in any way for their increased calorie intake for 100 days. Because 3,500 calories equals 1 pound of stored fat, these men should have each gained around 29 pounds in that time. However, some subjects with a high ability to convert calories to heat gained less than nine pounds, while others gained 29 pounds. The average weight gain was 18 pounds, which indicates most had some thermogenic effect.[1] Because activity levels were controlled, this study clearly shows the ability of some people to use their naturally high thermogenic activity—which cannot be externally controlled—to burn a large number of calories.

Many overweight people have reported that they do not sweat easily. Instead, their face turns beet red with exertion, but hardly any sweat appears or, if they are fit, it is hard to get their heart rate up to an aerobic level. This is all a part of being a super absorber. The body is hanging onto every fat particle it can, and not giving up much energy in proportion to effort expended. Fat people tend to fidget less than thin people do and sometimes avoid athletics because of social stigmas and difficulty in breathing upon exertion. They also tend to be less athletically inclined than their thinner counterparts.

Even though some may be genetically programmed to be heavy, almost every ethnicity will become fat if they live in

America. Europeans, Asians, African-Americans, Hispanics, Pacific Islanders, and East Indians are all more likely to become heavy in this country. America is a bad place to live if you do not want to be obese. Blame a food industry that wants your money and will "feed" you anything to get it.[2]

Brown Fat

Most of us have a mother, father, uncle or spouse who eats several candy bars a day, in addition to regular large meals with desserts and late night snacks, yet who still look like walking skeletons. These people may have larger amounts of "brown fat." Brown fat is a very enviable (but, alas, very rare) segment of fat that seems to have as its goal the burning of calories. Invisible to the naked eye, under a microscope it appears as fat laden with capillaries. Children are born with a high ratio of brown fat to white fat in comparison to adults. As we grow, the ratio changes gradually, so that most of us have very little brown fat left by the time we reach adulthood.

Genetics vs Lifestyle Choices

In some families, there is a lifestyle component to being heavy. In these families, rich meals and multiple snacks are the norm. Whether this is learned behavior, or a result of intrinsic hunger levels and genetic makeup, is unknown. It does seem that some people have an insatiable hunger level, while others are content with lesser amounts of food. Although this appears to be a lifestyle choice, it may simply be an inherited predisposition favoring the storage of fat.

Some people simply eat until their hunger has abated, and then stop; others eat whatever is available, whether or not they are hungry. In both cases, satiety signals seem to be based on genetic components related to serotonin levels in the brain, *and* to signals from different glands and organs in the body, such as the stomach, pancreas, hypothalamus and pineal glands. This difference is also noted in the animal kingdom: some mice and rats have a hearty willingness to eat all the food offered to them, while others do not eat once they are full, whether or not food is still available. This observed phenomenon suggests unhealthy eating habits are partially based on a genetic component.

The Importance of Small Changes

There may be a place for all those diet books after all. Certainly, the man or woman who has allowed 20 pounds or more to creep up over the last 20 years can benefit from more rigorous food control and exercise. An even better strategy is to change a few small habits that will result in slow (and more sustainable) weight loss over time. Increasing activity doesn't trigger the body to secrete more hunger hormones, as does dieting.

It has been said that giving up butter or margarine for a year will result in a 10-pound weight loss. Going up and down one additional flight of stairs per day will also result in a 10-pound weight loss a year. However, most of us want our weight lost yesterday, and are not willing to do something that involves such a long commitment, such as giving up butter or climbing the stairs at work every day. These strategies may lead to only a few pounds of weight loss each year, but they do add up, and result in lifestyle changes that improve overall health. The same people, who prefer a quick fix, may be surprised when they discover that the more diets they go on, the fatter they ultimately become.

According to Christiane Northrup, MD, bingeing may be a physiologically mandated behavior that occurs in direct proportion to the stringency of the diet we have been following.[3] Since weight generally comes off slowly and is regained rapidly, it follows that we will get fatter with each diet. However, for the genetically obese, *diets will never work.* How many diets do *you* have to fail on to finally discover this truth for yourself? Have you joined and rejoined a diet program several times? Have you lost and gained huge amounts of weight several times? Some obese people have lost 100 pounds five times over and are still fat. Some report having lost over 1,000 pounds in their life. The fact is, there are many successful dieters, but unfortunately, they are unable to maintain their weight loss because of biological forces that are not subject to willpower.

Small changes in eating habits will not put an end to their weight-gain. Many of these individuals cannot maintain a static weight. They report that, if they are not on a weight loss diet, they are gaining weight. Without constant control, these people will continue to gain until they reach their genetically predetermined weight (see Body Types on page 32). The weight of an older family member can often be an indicator of how the body will change with age, and what kind of weight-gains—or losses— might be expected. Other times, a genetic mutation may cause the person to become the first obese person in the family.

A man we'll call Jim is of normal weight, but has a family history of obesity. All of his eight brothers and sisters are obese. He eats very little, consuming about 1,500 calories a day, and only drinks distilled water. He plays racquetball several times a week, swims daily and exercises incessantly in order to stay thin. He does eat, but exhibits anorexic-like behavior, and is the father of an anorexic child. But, through total commitment and dedication to this one goal—staying thin—he has bucked his genetic destiny. Jim constantly monitors his fat intake, obsessively checks his weight, and exercises to get rid of what he perceives as excess fat. Not everyone is able to give this kind of dedication to staying thin; few people have either the time or the inclination.

Liposuction and Lipectomy

Many people, having failed at dieting, may opt to have the excess fat—on their bellies, hips, and thighs—surgically removed through processes called liposuction and lipectomy. It would seem logical that having fat cells vacuumed out, or cut off, not only offers an immediate solution to their weight problems, but also decreases their ability to gain weight. When cell size is decreased through diet or starvation, the brain stimulates a need to eat because the body wants to keep those fat cells at a certain size. However, it would appear that when the number of cells is decreased through removal, the brain also stimulates a need to eat since the body's natural tendency is to want to maintain cells at a certain *number,* and—contrary to old ideas—we *do* make more fat cells as adults. Moreover, having fat cells sucked out or cut off may be detrimental to overall health, depending on where in the body those cells are located. Early studies suggest that fat cells around the abdomen, especially visceral fat—deep fat surrounding the organs—can be harmful to overall health. Visceral fat cannot be sucked out or cut off, because it isn't just under the skin—it lies deep within the abdominal cavity.[4]

Unlike visceral fat, fat cells on the hips and thighs can be distinctly beneficial. It has been discovered that when fat cells are removed from the hips and thighs in women, the body becomes both glucose-intolerant and insulin–resistant, and that triglycerides increase. State University of New York Health Science Center surgeon John Kral removes 12 to 15 billion subcutaneous fat cells—10 and 13 pounds—from the hips and thighs of female patients, and found that afterward, the women's bodies were actually *less* effective at removing fat from the bloodstream, and *less* efficient at processing glucose. Dr. Kral also noted that, in his experience, extremely heavy women who have subcutaneous body fat surgically removed ultimately end up more apple than pear shaped.[5] They seem to have the health problems—high blood-fat levels, high blood pressure, diabetes and so on—that are associated with apple shapes. This was not the case with heavy women who retained their natural endowment of subcutaneous body fat in thighs and hips.

Faulty Studies

Many of the studies that point to obesity as a cause of increased mortality are flawed in some manner. For example: in 1975, 200 extremely heavy, but healthy, young men took part in a weight loss program at the VA Medical Center in Los Angeles. The men fasted and/or consumed a liquid diet for periods ranging from a month to two months. Each subject lost between 60 and 90 pounds. Over the next seven years, almost all of the men gained everything back, and more; *50 of the original 200 died.* This was a 25 percent mortality rate, or one in four. By contrast, mortality rates for men of similar age and weight would have resulted in only 11.2 out of 200 deaths.

This significant study showed that forced fasting and starvation caused a high percentage of death. The authors wrongly concluded that no factors other than obesity could have caused such mortality. However, other than their large size, the men had no acute health problems when first seen. That is, no problems *before losing weight*. It was only after the radical treatment that they started having problems—75 developed diabetes, 39 became hypertensive, 19 were diagnosed with cardiovascular disease, and 27 died of heart attacks.[6] Many studies blame obesity for illness and mortality rates, but most do not factor in the number of times a person has gained and lost weight as being part of the problem.

Hippocrates wrote about the dangers of dieting in 400 B.C.: "Dieting that causes excessive loss of weight...is beset with difficulties." Twenty-four hundred years later his warning is largely ignored. In the first anti-diet book, *Diet and Die* (1935), there were a few anecdotal stories about men and women who died while losing weight, or shortly after.[7] Seventy years of research since this book was published have produced a mountain of evidence about the hazards of chronic dieting and weight fluctuation. The real evidence shows that risks to health and longevity are more likely related to dieting, rather than from stable weights that are above those recommended by height-weight tables.[8]

Life Isn't Weighed on the Bathroom Scales

Before you begin yet another diet, consider seeking a gradual shift in perception that has meaning for you. This may very well give you the personal power you need to grow and learn the lessons of life. These paradigm shifts are suggested in the book *Life Isn't Weighed on the Bathroom Scales*.[9]

From	To
Willpower	Surrender to divine will
Beware of diets	Be aware of how diets affect you
Eating right as punishment	Eating right as learning discipline
Weight loss through science	Weight loss through grace
My body is defective	My body is trying to survive
Indulgence with food	Nurturance with food
I'll be happy when I'm thin	I might be thin once I'm happy
Need to control food	Trust in my inner wisdom
What's wrong with me?	What can I learn from this?
Am I being bad or good?	Am I empowered or diminished?
The goal is the victory	The journey holds the treasure
Eat to lose weight	Eat to feel healthy
Exercise to lose weight	Exercise to feel healthy
Fix me so I can be okay	I'm already okay and want to grow
I have a disease/character flaw	Weight as challenge and teacher
Victim	Warrior

Size-ism

Federal courts are beginning to recognize *size-ism*—discrimination against people who are extremely overweight. This recognition came when a Boston Federal Appeals Court, in a ruling that marked a first for the obese, extended disability rights to them in September 1993. The three-judge panel awarded a Rhode Island woman $100,000 after her employer told her that she could not return to work until she lost 117 pounds. The State of Rhode Island argued that her condition was not a handicap under anti-discrimination laws because it was self-inflicted. The

State was held liable because the Appeals Court interpreted that the law applies to many conditions that may possibly be voluntary, such as AIDS, cancer from cigarette smoking and diabetes. To win an obesity discrimination suit, there must be proof that the person suffers from long-term impairment that substantially limits major life activities.[10]

9

Measuring Obesity

Obesity is determined by the percentage of body fat in relation to the percentage of muscle. People might be over the limit for what would be considered "normal" weight but, if they are muscular, with a low percentage of body fat, they are not obese. Others might be normal or underweight, but have excessive body fat.

New guidelines use three key measures to determine whether a person is overweight: body mass index (BMI); waist circumference; risk factors for diseases and conditions associated with obesity.

Body Mass Index

According to some, the current best single gauge for body fat is a measurement called body mass index (BMI). BMI is determined by multiplying a person's weight in pounds by 703, and then dividing the result twice by their height in inches.

For example, a woman who weighs 150 pounds and is 68 inches tall would have a BMI of 22.8.

150 x 703 = 105,450
105,450 ÷ 68 = 1,550.74
1,550.77 ÷ 68 = 22.8

The result is compared to a printed chart that indicates levels of body fat. However, this method is not perfect because it does not measure levels of fitness.

Guidelines currently define *obese* as a BMI of 30 or greater. Studies indicate that the lowest risks for heart disease, diabetes and some cancers are found in people with a BMI of 21 to 25. The risks increase slightly if values are between 25 to 27. They are considered significant between 27 to 30, and dramatic if over 30.[1]

The American Society for Bariatric Surgery classifies levels of obesity according to the following table:

Method of classifying levels of obesity:

Rating	BMI	Estimated Extra Pounds
Normal BMI	<25	0 pounds overweight
Overweight	25 to 27	0 to 20
Mild Obesity	27 to 30	20 to 50
Moderate Obesity	30 to 35	50 to 75
Severe Obesity	35 to 40	75 to 100
Morbid Obesity	40 to 50	100 to 200
Super Obesity	50 to 60	200+

While the BMI is a useful index, levels of fitness can vary. For example, a superb male athlete may weigh 210 pounds at 6 feet tall; his BMI by this formula would be the same as a couch potato with a beer belly at the same weight and height. (BMI = 28) Clearly one has more muscle mass and one more fat mass.

Waist Circumference

New guidelines note that abdominal fat is very important in assessing risk of disease. One study suggested that women whose waistlines are over 35 inches, and men whose waists measure over 40 inches, are at increased risk for heart disease, diabetes, and impaired functioning. A more precise indication of risk is the distribution of body fat around the chest, and upper hips, as well as around the abdomen. The distribution of fat can be evaluated by dividing waist size by hip size. For example, a women with a 30-inch waist and 40-inch hips would have a ratio of .75; one with a 41-inch waist and 39-inch hips would have a ratio of 1.05, and be considered an apple shape. The lower the ratio, the better. The risk of heart disease rises sharply for women whose ratios are over .8, and for men with ratios over 1.0.[2] This ratio also gives an indication of the amount of a person's deep visceral fat (fat within the abdominal cavity itself, discussed in Chapter 8).

Determining Body Fat Percentage

The only precise way to measure body fat is with underwater weighing. This method is cumbersome and not widely available to most people.[3] Scales that claim to measure body fat are based on the premise that a small charge of electricity going through the body will travel faster through the lean mass than the fat mass (bioelectrical impedance analysis). They give a rough percentage of body fat and perhaps more importantly, measure changes in the percentage over time.

Metabolic Regulation of Weight

The adipostat, located in the hypothalamus gland within the brain, dictates the level of fat in the body. This mechanism acts like a thermostat, and seeks to maintain a genetically determined body weight. It establishes a set-point that changes over time, usually rising with age. The brain maintains this pre-established goal by regulating the expenditure or storage of energy, until stored fat meets the level determined by the adipostat.

Losing weight, when the adipostat is trying to maintain or increase it, is remarkably difficult. It would be like trying to stay warm in an ice-cold room. Soon you would be compelled to turn up the heat. In the same way, your adipostat compels you to eat in order to remain comfortable. Most dieters don't realize that the brain is undermining their weight loss efforts by working to obtain the body's original weight. It does this by activating the sensation of hunger more often, by slowing the metabolism, or by reducing motivation to exercise to offset calorie loss. The adipostat can be slightly reset for lower fat stores only by maintaining healthy eating and regular, vigorous exercise over a long period of time.

Genetic Factors

We have learned that there are a number of ways that genetics play a major role in weight control: the location of fat on the body, metabolic rates, food preferences (some people like salty foods, others prefer sweets), hormone regulation and hunger levels are some of the genetic factors that were formerly thought to be environmental. The human metabolism evolved over time so that it could conserve energy and store fat for times of famine. Most mild-to-moderate obesity currently occurs in people with normal physiology who eat too much and exercise too little.

Some experts think that type II diabetes is actually a gene, developed thousands of years ago, that regulated insulin resistance so that in the winter, when food supplies were low, storing food as body fat was easier.

Some genetic mutations have been recently discovered. One appears to increase the number and size of fat cells and is associated with super obesity. The melanocortin-4 gene receptor, which plays a key role in shutting off the urge to eat, is defective in some families with a history of obesity. Another gene mutation is called POMC. It affects several different hormones, and produces a combination of obesity, red hair, and deficiencies in stress hormones. One small study found evidence of a previous infection by an organism called adenovirus Ad-36 in obese people, but not in lean people. These genetic markers indicate that there are several genes responsible for obesity. The presence of a greater number of them predisposes certain people to obesity.

10

Healthy Attitudes

The biggest problem with diets is staying on them. With most diets, you *do* lose weight if you follow the plan. However, it is difficult to stay on any diet for a long time, especially if you have been on more than a few. It is even more difficult to maintain the weight loss once you go off the diet. In the long run, sensible eating plans work better than dieting. The Uniformed Services University enrolled 24 overweight women in a 13-week study. All went to group meetings with a psychologist, and began walking for 30 minutes three times a week. Half were put on a traditional low-fat diet of 1,200 calories a day, with high-calorie foods off-limits.

The other 12 women, armed with meal plans and recipes, followed an easier regimen that allowed 1,800 calories per day. Many of them felt that they were eating too much food. At the group sessions, counselors encouraged these women to forget dieting rules and to accept themselves, regardless of their weight. The women also learned to dine in moderation. If someone had an urge for a particular food, say potato chips, they were allowed to have 20, instead of a whole bag. The goal was to teach them not to diet, but to develop a way of eating that they could stick to for the rest of their lives.

As expected, those on the low-calorie diet lost more weight in the 13 weeks than the healthy eaters, 12 pounds to 5. But, one year later, the non-dieters had dropped a total of 22 pounds and the dieters had gained back three. So the overall effect on the strict dieters was a total loss of nine pounds and, on the sensible eaters, 22 pounds. In addition, the sensible eaters had changed some habits that encouraged continued weight loss and health, while the dieters had gone back to the old habits that had led to their weight-gain in the first place.[1]

It is very difficult to eat in a restricted way for long periods of time because the body has built-in defenses against losing weight. The body interprets dieting as starvation, and both psychological and biological forces work against it after a while. While the less radical healthy eating approach will not make you model-thin, learning to listen to and honor your body's wants can enhance weight loss efforts.

Insulin Resistance

Good metabolism means that your body maximizes the chemical processes within it, and minimizes the risk of disease. Insulin is a hormone that enables your body to utilize the food you eat. Whenever you eat a meal with carbohydrates, glucose levels (also called blood sugar levels) in your blood rise. Glucose circulates through the bloodstream, where most of your cells are unable to use it until insulin arrives. The cells are "locked," and insulin is the key that opens the lock to allow them to use the glucose. The more glucose in the blood, the more insulin is released—and the more glucose can be used.

In the best cases, your cells are "insulin-sensitive" and do as they are told, getting the glucose into the muscles and liver, and storing it there until your body needs it for energy. Sometimes this process is not "on duty," and cells can't utilize insulin. Cells that act as though they are locked against insulin are called insulin-resistant cells. About one-quarter of the United States population has cells that are insulin resistant, ranging from mildly reactive to almost inert. When insulin resistance develops, it doesn't affect all cells equally. Rather, the cells that display the highest resistance are those in the muscles and liver, which happen to be the most important organs for processing glucose. In the meantime, while too much insulin is collecting in the bloodstream, the fat that a person eats is entering the existing fat cells without having to have insulin to unlock those cells. So, consumed fat goes into fat cells, and the glucose and insulin levels are not used efficiently for metabolism.

Some studies have shown that increased insulin levels also lead to increased hunger for sugary foods. In other words, the more sugar you eat, the more you want. If cells continue to be insulin resistant, over the course of many years the person may eventually develop full-fledged type II diabetes. This occurs only after a long, slow process of deterioration, and is why adult-onset diabetes is usually detected only in middle age. The body deals with the problem of insulin resistance by forcing the pancreas to pump out more insulin, and to bombard the cells with an overload. However, this only makes the critical cells more resistant to utilizing glucose judiciously. The result is increased insulin resistance.[2]

Causes of insulin resistance include a sedentary lifestyle and a high-fat, high-sugar diet. These two factors are also at fault for excess weight. Insulin is a very powerful stimulator for fat storage. The more unused insulin there is in the body, the greater the likelihood that the body will store fat. Thus, even if a person does not eat too much, *he is likely to get fatter* if he is insulin resistant.

What can be done to counteract insulin resistance? The answer is mild to moderate exercise several times a week, along with reduced fat and sugar in the diet. A study of males who had trained for at least 5 years and had run 10 or more miles every week, showed that insulin resistance was not a problem. Older (70 years plus) and middle-aged (ages 40 to 69) athletes had increased insulin sensitivity in active muscles, and improved vascularization (blood flow) to active tissues.[3] They used glucose effectively for energy and did not easily store fat.

Exercise Decreases Insulin Resistance

The minimum recommended amount of exercise is 10 minutes of moderate exercise at least 15 times each week. For further information on recommended fitness regimens, see the "Spark" program in the book *The Spark: The Revolutionary 3-Week Plan that Changes Everything You Know About Exercise, Weight Control and Health.*[4] The biggest factor in counteracting insulin resistance seems to be the amount and intensity of exercise. Even if a person consumes calories over their recommended limit, exercise and a diet rich in complex carbohydrates seem to ensure weight stabilization and/or loss. More importantly, the body is no longer resistant to insulin nor prone to overweight (even though the person had been eating fewer calories than naturally thin people). This is because the body has a very hard time converting complex carbohydrates into fat. Carbohydrates tend to get used immediately for energy, not stored, and even when they *are* stored, they are stored in muscle tissue, and not easily converted to fat.

At the Osaka University Medical School, 15 very large professional Sumo wrestlers were studied. Each had an average BMI of 36—way over the cutoff point for obesity—consumed 5,000 to 7,000 calories per day, and exercised strenuously for several hours every day. Despite their obvious obesity, these wrestlers had very little visceral (inner) body fat, as assessed by CAT scans. They also had low levels of cholesterol and blood glucose.[5] The moral seems to be that if you're going to eat a lot, then be sure to exercise a lot, too.

One study in the *American Journal of Clinical Nutrition* found that it was virtually impossible to gain weight on a high-carbohydrate, low-fat diet. At the University of Illinois at Chicago, 18 women between the ages of 20 and 48, with BMIs ranging from 18 to 44, consumed a diet consisting of 20 percent fat for a period of 20 weeks, so that researchers could assess its impact on weight and body fat. Before the diet, the women's average fat intake was 37 percent. During the course of the 20 weeks, the nutritionists kept adjusting the food intake upward, to see how much could be consumed without resulting in weight-gain. Not only was there no weight-gain, but they could not prevent weight loss, even though the women were consuming an average of 27,000 calories more than their usual intake during a comparable time. By the concluding week, the women were eating 350 more calories per day, but were losing weight. Despite eating more than 41,000 extra calories over the 20 weeks—which should have caused them to gain 11.7 pounds—the six women who initially weighed the most lost an average of 4.5 pounds.[6]

On the diet, the women were consuming *more* calories, but 26 *fewer* grams of fat per day. How many fat grams does that translate into each day? For most women, it would mean consuming somewhere between 44 to 50 grams of fat per day—instead of the usual 70 to 100 grams seen in diets heavy in fats and fast foods. A quarter-pound hamburger can have as many as 40-plus grams of fat. If combined with french fries and a shake, you would be consuming more fat in one meal than is needed in a day. For men, between 60 to 70 grams of fat would put them in the 20 to 25 percent fat consumption figure.

"Set" Weight

If a man consumes an average of 2,500 calories per day, he will consume over 1,000,000 calories in a year. If the man's weight remains stable, we can assume that the number of calories he burns would exactly match the number he consumes. It is most unlikely, however, that there would be such a perfect match between input and output. Suppose that the difference between the two was only 1 percent more calories taken in than calories burned. This would add up to 10,000 calories—or about 3 pounds of body fat—per year. If this imbalance continued unchecked, it would result in a gain of 30 pounds per decade, or more than 150 pounds of weight-gain over the course of 50 years.

Most men, however, do not go from an average weight of 150 to over 300 pounds between the ages of 20 to 70. There is clearly some mechanism within each of us that works to "set" our body weight at a certain point, and to maintain it at a reasonably constant level over long periods of time. How that works, and why it varies so much from person to person is a mystery. We can only assume that "set" weight is probably genetic (see Genetic Factors on page 117).[7]

Weight-gain in infants is another story. A baby who weighs 7 pounds at birth will typically double his or her weight in the first four months of life. If an infant consumes and average of six ounces of mother's milk six times a day, he will have consumed approximately 480 calories per day for 120 days. Since each pound of weight is equal to about 3,500 calories, that baby will have taken in 57,600 calories—equal to almost 17 pounds. But most babies do not weigh anywhere near 24 pounds at four months; they are closer to 14 pounds. What became of the other 10 pounds that we would expect them to have gained from all those calories? They were burned in their brown fat stores (see page 105), and affected by thermogenics (see page 103). Whether the baby is active and cries, or is passive and sleeps most of the time, the expected weight-gain can be charted with accuracy.

Most of us also consume more calories than we burn. However, we are not blessed with an infant's high percentage (5 percent) of brown fat—fat that is known to burn excess calories. Consequently, an adult's activity level has a big effect on the number of calories stored and/or burned.

A Different Attitude

The thoughts that lead some people to believe that they are less worthy as human beings than others, because of the way they look, are negative. Continually obsessing about the way we look leads to a loss of self-identity because we are never satisfied. This also wastes time and energy that could be spent more productively. By setting aside our quest for thinness, we can find happiness pursuing other things of value—our family, our relationships, and our inner selves—without distraction. An equally productive goal would be to be fit at any weight.

The fear of not being accepted because of being fat leads us to act in ways that make it hard for people to connect to us. A slender news reporter wanted to find out what it was like to be fat in today's society, so she donned a "fat suit" and went out for a day in New York City. Just as she had expected, people were rude to her, and she got shoddier treatment at department stores than she customarily received as a thin person—she felt ridiculed. But was it because she expected this treatment, and therefore subtly attracted it? By way of contrast, a confident naturally fat person could spend the same day in New York, ride on the same bus, and go to the same store without feeling the least bit ridiculed, or being mistreated at the department store. The difference for the reporter may have been her own attitude about herself as a fat person. People tend to treat us the way we expect them to

Our expectations usually have more to do with our attitudes and actions toward others, rather than with their attitudes toward us. Generally speaking, we share the responsibility for the way we are treated. As philosopher C. T. Warner says, "It is our attitude toward others—it is the way we see them—that gives them provocation and excuse for doing what we are blaming them for. This principle can be addressed in the brief maxim: 'Seeing other people as the problem IS the problem'."[8]
A heavy person with a great attitude and personality is a joy to know, and can overcome stereotypes through his or her own "Wonderful Me" demeanor.

Oprah Winfrey is a good role model. Her audience has witnessed her weight change repeatedly over the years—from quite heavy, to exceptionally slim, and finally to average. Because of her engaging personality and interest in others, the weight does not matter. In fact, it makes her more approachable, more human.

Putting it to the Test

The following section is from the book, *Making Peace with the Image in the Mirror,* by Steven R. Hawks, PhD.[9]

Some years ago, Steve (my biologist coworker) and I were at a conference in Washington, D.C. As we traveled on the subway system, we became engaged in a deep discussion... "Isn't it interesting," I commented, "that even though there is a universal need for love and acceptance, virtually every passenger on this subway seems to be in their own isolated world—even while being surrounded by thousands and millions of fellow travelers."

"What would happen," Steve asked, "if, instead of worrying about what others may or may not be thinking about us, we were to focus our energies on noticing those people around us, and then express our sincere perceptions to them?"

After debating this question for some time, we decided to seek an answer in the form of an experiment or, rather, a contest. The rules of the contest were simple:

(a) Focus your attention on a fellow subway rider and form a sincere, positive perception in relation to that person.

(b) Express your perception to him or her in an open and honest manner.

(c) Take notice of the response. No response or a negative response was worth zero points. A smile or kind response was worth 10, a handshake was worth 20, and a pat on the arm

was worth 30. A response that took the form of a hug earned an immediate 50 points, while a kiss brought in an automatic 100.

My first traveler was an older woman standing nearby, whose unfocused gaze was directed out a darkened window. After turning my full attention on her, I approached and said, "Excuse me, but your hat reminds me of one that my sister likes to wear. Do you mind telling me about it?" At first, she was somewhat startled at the intrusion but, once she sensed that my question was sincere, she provided me with the natural history of her hat as requested. We then spoke of my sister's hat and how much it meant to her. Our discussion moved on to general topics of family, a declaration of common interests, and finally to an expression of delight at having met and shared some moments together.

I was left with a tender pat on the arm as she stepped off the train at her stop.

Steve and I became so intrigued and enthusiastic with our contest that it lasted for much of the day as we visited the Smithsonian museums, strolled about the Mall, and returned to the hotel on the subway. We visited with people of all ages, both sexes, many different races, and many nationalities. We both brought in more than 1,000 points.

Before we were finished, our small contest had yielded many

insights. The most important was that, since people are bur-
dened with worry about how they are being perceived by others,
the unsolicited expression of a sincere, positive perception is
received most gladly. It generally led to lively discussions,
mutual manifestations of warmth and kindness and, in the
end, to a very friendly parting of the ways (with even a few
hugs). And yet, most subway riders stare vacantly ahead, read
a book, or sleep—often preoccupied with wonder about what
others might be thinking of them, but never once forming or
expressing a perception they might have developed of someone
else. And thus the loneliness and isolation overwhelm us, while
meaningful companionship is only an arm' length away. If
only we could overcome the fear of rejection and be the one to
step forward first.

This experiment was important because it shows that to be accepted as a person is more important than how a person looks. As one philosopher said, "If another person only had in his storehouse of deserved self-esteem what you had put there, what would he have to draw upon to sustain him?"[10]

The Need for Love and Acceptance

The leading cause of depression among married women is loneliness and lack of romance.[11] What happens to you if no one ever expresses love to you? What if you are single, or involved with someone totally insensitive to your needs? How do you get others to like you? Do you spend the rest of your life trying to find the love you feel you deserve in any way you can? Or do you eat to fill the void?

We cannot control how other people feel about us. That is true whether we are fat or thin. Other people cannot be depended on to fulfill our need for love and acceptance. That does not mean that our need goes away. If we look to others for approval, we may spend the rest of our lives stuck in unfulfilled misery.[12]

Take the example of Forrest Gump, in the movie of the same name. Forrest loves Jenny, and shows her in many ways how devoted he is to her. However, Jenny does not return his love. After she leaves, he writes to her faithfully, but all the letters are returned. Finally, after many years of drugs, promiscuity, and disappointments, Jenny runs out of options and returns to Alabama. She stays with Forrest while she tries to recover from her past. Then Forrest proposes to her and tells her he would make a good husband. "Yes," Jenny answers, "you would make a good husband, Forrest."

"But you won't marry me," says Forrest. But this time Forrest has the last word. "I am not a smart man, but I know what love is."

For Jenny, love was all about how *she* felt. It was the attention from others, the audiences she sang to, or her less-than-ideal boyfriends. But, in the end, they all abandoned her. For Forrest, love was undying devotion and commitment to the welfare of another person, no matter how she treated him or what she did with her life. His love was constant and unfaltering. He had no facades or false pretenses. He wasn't worried about rejection. Even though love was not expressed to him, he met his need for love by feeling and expressing it for someone else.

Steven R. Hawks, a noted nutritionist and health advisor said, "The first step to filling our lives with love and acceptance is not to be loved by others, but to develop feelings of love for others, and then to express that love to them in the form of devoted commitment to their welfare and happiness. Whether

others accept or reject the love that we offer has greater impli-
cations for them than for us."[13]

Being focused outward rather than inward is the best way to
overcome the negative feelings we have about our own appearance. The more we forget about ourselves, the more time there
is to do something worthwhile in the world.

11

Personal Stories

A study of former bariatric patients was begun using the Internet to solicit opinions and personal stories about weight loss surgery. This survey was undertaken to present both sides of the weight loss surgery issue.

Numerous bariatric doctors around the world are performing this surgery without adequately preparing or following up with their patients, while other doctors are committed to supporting and following their patients. The advertising techniques some doctors employ are questionable because of their one-sided presentation. Virtually all of the results that a person is likely to see when given a video or live presentation produced by the bariatric surgeon are positive. The negative ramifications are not discussed at length, and are glossed over as if they are few and inconsequential. The overweight person is primed to see the positive and dismiss the negative because they want a similar outcome. It's akin to a financial seminar in which a presenter has a hot commodity that is "sure" to make money. The reality, that you could lose everything, is thought to be preposterous—until it happens. The realities of weight loss surgery are often to be found in the support groups and Internet chat rooms with people who have had the surgery.

Although side effects are mentioned, the actual reality of changing one's total relationship with food is not fully absorbed by the participants. Many people are pulled into having the surgery, never having heard a negative report of any kind about it

There are only a few essential ingredients to life: air, sleep, water, shelter, and food. Taking food away and replacing normal hunger and eating patterns with artificially small meals, boring high-protein shakes, and a multitude of vitamin and mineral pills, has the potential to devastate a person's health and vitality.

The demands placed on individuals by society to conform to acceptable size requirements are also harmful. My conclusion is that weight loss surgery has a place for the extremely heavy person who also has fundamental health issues to deal with. Other people who wish to lose weight should do so by making incrementally small behavioral adjustments and adding exercise and movement to their day. The concept of repeatedly dieting to lose a great amount of weight quickly (yo-yo dieting) seems to be flawed, with more health problems appearing because of its cumulative effects on the body.

This survey asked for the respondents' experiences with weight loss surgery, both positive and negative. Twenty-three of the stories were selected for this book because of their unique and varied accounts. Most of those who had positive experiences reported the basic premise that they were very happy: They were happy to have had the surgery and would do it again because they were now thin; whereas before the surgery, they had little hope.

The case histories that follow reflect the overall statistical findings of the 132 original respondents: two-thirds of them experienced significant weight loss; two-thirds of the 132 were women. (Photos included in the book do not coincide with the stories. They were solicited just prior to the book's publication, while the survey was conducted in 2000.)

Since weight loss surgery almost always results in weight loss, and only a very small percentage drop out, reverse the procedure, or do not have the expected outcome, the results are skewed in such a way that a graph of weight loss is meaningless. For example, if most start at one body size (fat) and end at another body size (thin) one would infer that the process is linear: Be fat, get the surgery, become thin.

That doesn't tell the whole story; in fact, it barely scratches the surface. It would be like saying that one is born, lives a life and then dies, experiences notwithstanding. In writing about these people, I hoped to describe the different experiences people have had in undergoing a radical surgery that severely alters the digestive system.

People with psychological problems will discover it does not change the basic tenants of one's life, and happiness cannot be purchased at the hands of a surgeon. Overweight people who have this surgery with the wrong expectations can become even more miserable after the surgery. It changes the way they relate to food, one of the essentials of life, in a basic and unchangeable way. If patients had previously used food for psychological support, comfort, stuffing of feelings, or other unhealthy habits, then the surgery may exacerbate those original problems by creating new ones.

Weight loss surgery doesn't transform a miserable life into an extraordinarily happy one. Sophia Williams, a counselor involved in changing people's perceptions about themselves said, "Wherever you go and whatever you do, you take yourself." [1]

The stories that follow present both everyday and extreme circumstances that have occurred after having one of the weight loss surgeries.

---

1. Williams, Sophia. Minority Women and Self Esteem. City University, Tacoma, WA. Dissertation 1995. u.p.

Bill

My name is Bill, and I had the bileopancreatic diversion (BPD) surgery a few months ago. I haven't had such a great experience with it. I don't think I was ready for the life style changes it required. I chose the most radical of all the surgeries because I was tired of being overweight, and I didn't want to continue with my life if I had to be fat. I started out weighing 425 pounds. I come from a family of thin people, and I had always been the one they couldn't figure out. My dad kept looking for reasons why I was heavy; maybe it was my disdain for sports. They didn't realize I hated sports because it was hard to fit into the uniforms, hard to run, and hard to excel at anything I tried. That was what turned me off of sports. No matter how I did, there was always someone in my family that could do it better, including my mom.

Immediately after coming out of surgery, my temperature spiked up to 105°F, and I was rushed back into the operating room. Apparently I had sprung a "leak," and stomach contents were leaking out into my abdominal cavity. After undergoing a second operation on the same day, I was pretty wasted. I felt shaky and sweaty in recovery, and the feeling didn't go away for several days. I couldn't get enough of the pain medication. I kept ringing for the nurse, and she kept telling me I couldn't have anymore for one or two more hours. I felt like screaming, and I did holler at the nurses quite a bit. I wanted to get up off the bed, rip out my IV and put a gun to my head. I felt uneasy and anxious. After they took out the esophageal tube, I did lots of moaning and groaning. I know I was a pain to be around, but I didn't care. I just wanted the wonderful part that I had been expecting to start. After the first day in the hospital I sprung another leak. I was rushed in for more surgery.

At that point I thought I had done the wrong thing. I no longer trusted my doctor and I was ready to die. Having three doses of anesthesia in 26 hours and three surgeries—two of them because my life was hanging in the balance—was grim. Besides that, my doctor seemed to think that I was in some way responsible. He kept telling me I would have to calm down and not get so agitated. He switched pain medications and, for some reason, that helped a lot. I think I had a reaction to the Percocet that caused me to get agitated and sweaty whereas, with most people, it calms them down. I was getting a morphine drip at that point. I had control over the flow, and I felt a lot better being able to control my own dosage of medication. I always gave myself more than I thought I needed because I didn't want to feel bad again. I began to have tremendous bouts of gastrointestinal distress and gas. Sometimes the nurses would try to air the room out before they would come in. My roommate asked to be moved, and I don't blame him. Besides the smell, the cramps in my stomach were horrendous. I could sometimes see the skin rise up on one side of my abdomen and spasm on the other. It felt like a storm was raging inside my gut. The only thing I looked forward to were the ice chips to suck on. Food turned me off.

After four days, I was able to go home. I didn't think I was ready, and I was right, but they shoved me out the door anyway. Once at home, a black depression came on. I wanted my wife to bring me some pudding, cake, or some doughnuts, but instead I could only drink some putrid tasting protein drink, and water. I was supposed to get up and move around a little every day, but I preferred to stay in bed. I had my wife bring me a soda can to pee in because in I was so lethargic. Then she would have to empty it, and it was gross for her. I was pretty cleaned out, so I didn't have a bowel movement for several days.

I wouldn't let my wife turn off the light at night because I was sure, if she did, I would fall asleep and then I would die. It was irrational because I wanted to die but, on the other hand, I wouldn't let myself die. I hadn't really slept for several days and was starting to hallucinate. By this time I was having some unusual swelling around the incision, and some bloating. My wife suggested that by staying in bed I had let the fluids pool in my abdomen, and she recommended I get up and get dressed. She finally called the doctor; he ordered an ambulance to take me back to the hospital. I guess my refusal to get out of bed was threatening my life and I was at risk for developing an embolism, and I was encouraging the swelling.

In the hospital, the physical therapists came by and demanded that I get up and get moving. It hurt a great deal at first to just dangle my legs over the side of the bed. I would be huffing and puffing within 10 minutes of exertion. Over the next four days, they gradually got me out of bed and walking down the hall a bit. When I could manage going to the bathroom by myself and also wanted to take a shower, they recommended that I be sent home. This time I didn't just get a handout of instructions, but the doctor came by in person. He kept stressing the importance of getting up out of bed for several hours a day, and also told me I needed to shower, shave, and get dressed.

I thought he was again blaming me for my poor outcome and I felt resentful. However, this time I felt better when I went home and I was able to follow his advice. Gradually, over the next few weeks, I began to feel better. It was especially nice to turn in size 56 pants that I had belted to stay up, for a 48. I hadn't weighed myself at all since the surgery because I was afraid I had only lost 20 or 30 pounds. I had done that on other diets and then started gaining back the weight. I was pleasantly surprised when I stepped on the scale one month after my surgery to see I had lost over 40 pounds. This was more than I had lost in recent years and it didn't seem to be slowing down. I was soon into size 44 pants and then, to my amazement, a size 40. By this time I had lost over 100 pounds in less than four months. I then weighed 325 pounds and began to get motivated to go to the gym again. I hadn't been for a long, long time because of the stares I got and the looks of disapproval.

I no longer have to move my entire body from side to side when I walk in order to get my knees past each other. My wife used to call me a lumbering giant. Now I feel like an athlete. I knew men who wore jeans with a size 40 on the label on the outside, something not to be ashamed of. To me, they looked normal. I couldn't believe I was of normal size.

The doctor recommended I go back for stomach reconstruction. I'm considering it. I do have some flabby skin on my stomach, but I'm not sure I want to go under the knife again anytime soon. I also have halitosis that I can't seem to get rid of, and I have to take a lot of supplements every day.

Looking back, I can see that I did contribute somewhat to my poor surgical experience and recovery. I think I needed a counselor to help me through the rough spots. I recognize that I fell into a deep depression following my surgery—partly due to complications, partly to mismanagement of drugs and partly due to my fears. Now that I'm hovering around 200 pounds and have a size 38 waist, I feel great about myself. My wife is happy with me once again, now that I'm up and going to work and helping her around the house.

She really had it bad there for a while when I was being such a baby. I can't understand why she didn't scream at me or jab a knife in my chest at night when I wouldn't go to sleep and wouldn't let her turn out the light. She was left to take care of the house, the kids, my needs, and to still try to keep her sanity for several weeks. I can't thank her enough for staying with me and supporting me through this very difficult ordeal.

Fatimah

I don't think I was truly meant to be overweight. Sometimes I think if I'd never gotten pregnant, I wouldn't be overweight. However, some time after the birth of my twins, I realized I weighed as much as I had when nine months pregnant. I wonder if I would still be at that weight—which was less than 185 pounds—if I hadn't gone on all the diets. We are well-off, and so I joined the spa, went to summer retreats for fat people, tried every diet, and even injections of sheep urine, to try to lose weight.

In college and high school I had been an athlete. I loved playing tennis and swimming, and I won awards. Then, after the kids were old enough to try sports for themselves, I was busy shuttling them around and watching them play. I began to pile on the weight. It seemed like every new diet I tried put more weight on me. Finally, I was 150 pounds over what the weight tables said I should weigh. I should weigh around 150 pounds, because I'm fairly tall, and I weighed 300. Our scale actually only went up to 300, and I refused to get weighed at the doctor's offices after that. When they would tell me to jump up on the scale, I would tell the attendant to write down 300 pounds. I didn't want to be depressed the rest of the day by what I saw on the scale. I could barely survive knowing it was 300 pounds.

I saw an ad on the TV about the bariatric treatment center. Since the center was four hours away, I dismissed that idea. However, the idea kept coming back to me. The people on the video I ordered seemed to haunt me in my dreams. They were fat and now they were thin. It seemed magical. Some of them didn't even look like the same person. Other companies that advertised for the formerly fat never showed people five or ten years after their diets. These people who had weight loss surgery were still thin long after that.

One day I shared the video with my husband. I told him I wasn't going to do it because the center was too far away. He said he'd support whatever decision I made. I decided to go for a consultation. Since then, my dreams have come true. My friend, Liz, who is a size 10, said she'd go with me for the surgery. My husband was put in charge of things at home. My friend and I had always wanted to get away for a girl's-only weekend retreat. This wasn't quite what we'd had in mind, but Liz was a trouper. She stayed in my room and slept in a chair for two nights.

The morning of my surgery, my friend gave me a package. In it was a gorgeous safari suit, complete with hat and boots. It was a size eight. That was seven sizes smaller than what I wore at that time, which was a 22. I held it up and laughed with joy at the thought that someday I might fit into such a tiny outfit. At the time, the waistband fit over one thigh.

I breezed through the surgery and had only minor discomfort. I was on my way home two days later and felt great the whole way. However, a few days later, I developed a tender spot that turned out to be a seroma. That happens when some bacteria gets into the wound and causes an infection. It was a lump of pus right under the incision. I had to have it opened up and drained several times a day for a week. That was annoying, but not really a big complication of the surgery. The biggest concern I had was foul-smelling gas, but it went away about four months after my surgery. It took about 18 months to lose the 150 pounds. The first 100 came off within the first six months, and then it took another year to lose the remaining 50. I went back for reconstructive surgery on my flabby stomach that took away all the hanging skin. My final weight, where I have been for over two years, is 142 pounds.

When I finally got to my goal weight, I put on my safari suit and told my husband we were going to Africa that summer. He was delighted and promptly put it on his calendar. I've never been happier. Liz and I finally got to take our dream vacation together without kids and without husbands. It was great to put on a smaller size than my skinny friend and go out to the pool with her. I'm back to the person I'm supposed to be. I don't know why I got fat. I think it was all the diets, or maybe the stress of controlling my eating according to someone else's plan. I know I don't plan to let it happen again.

Tom

I was only 40 years old and weighed over 500 pounds. I didn't have a life. I stayed in my easy chair most nights after my seated job doing data entry. That's when my doctor told me that, because of my extremely high blood pressure (190/120), I wouldn't make it many more years if I didn't do something about my weight. My father had been obese, and had died at age 52—so I knew he was telling the truth. I had married young and we had two great children. However, I was unable to go with them to most school and church functions. I couldn't always be sure the chairs provided would hold me. I didn't even think of going into a restaurant—partly because I couldn't fit into a booth, and partly because of the looks I got from people. I knew how devastated I was when my father died while I was in college, and I didn't want my children to have to go through that.

I saw a commercial on TV for the surgical treatment of obesity and felt chills go up and down my spine. I immediately knew that this was the only way I would ever get the weight off. I have gone up and down the scale numerous times. I lost over 200 pounds once on TOPS (Take Off Pounds Sensibly), but it—plus another 100 pounds—had come back since then. I was tired of always feeling tired. I remembered having energy at one time, but now my life consisted of work, TV, eating, and sleeping. I tuned out my wife and the kids, and was turning into a recluse. I couldn't get life insurance because of my risk factors. However, when I was thinner, I had gotten a $150,000 policy. I often wondered if my family wouldn't be better off with the money than with such a blimp for a dad. I never felt happy, but couldn't seem to get motivated enough to do another diet. There were just too many failures associated with dieting.

It took just over four months to get surgery approved by my insurance company. I had the bypass gastroplasty that is somewhat like the old stomach stapling, but with the small intestine redone. I had to pay for 20 percent of the cost. That was about $5,000. I would've paid for it all. The doctor told me it would be a risky operation because of my weight and blood pressure. I had to sign a waiver releasing him from liability if I died from the surgery.

I went in at 7:00 A.M. on March 7, 1999. The IV was started immediately, and I was given something to drink that didn't taste too swell. After that I think I must have been given relaxants because I don't remember much more. I was in the recovery room by about 2:00 P.M., and vaguely remember hearing the words, "Everything went fine." Then I was in and out of consciousness for several more hours.

I woke up with unbelievable pain at about 11:00 that night and screamed for anyone to "help me." I was shown how to use a self-monitored pain dispenser. The pain subsided somewhat and I was able to sleep. I remember thinking, "I'm still alive," and not being too sure that that was a good thing. I had the dry heaves much of the time and nothing would go through the outlet. The worst thing that happened to me was that I began to vomit blood. They did an endoscopy and balloon dilation because my outlet froze shut and nothing was getting through. Then, while they were doing that, something tore—the lining or something—and it was very scary for a while. Before I left for home they did another balloon dilation and endoscopy to make sure the outlet wasn't too small. That is uncomfortable but not really painful, because they drug you.

Over the next few days I had to get out of bed and get moving. They don't just let you lie in bed, because muscles atrophy and there is increased risk for clots. By the time I went home, five days later, I was feeling pretty good. So far, I had just been given liquids to drink. The last day I tried some mashed up fruit in yogurt, and some mashed potatoes. I was able to eat about two bites of each at separate meals. I was extremely hungry for regular food. They put a vomit basin by me, but I never actually threw up. I did get dry heaves sometimes but, for some reason, the food just wouldn't come up.

At home, I convalesced for about two weeks. I mostly slept, but then caught up on some reading and bugged my wife incessantly for something else to do, because I was bored. She had been making an afghan; she told me to finish it for her and showed me how to crochet. My stitches apparently weren't very good compared to hers, so she took mine apart and bought me some yarn of my own to make my own afghan. I crocheted an afghan during the next month. I never thought I would admit that to anyone, but it was good therapy to make something nice.

I went back to work for half days starting the third week. I do computer work and so it wasn't demanding physically. After one month I was back to driving myself to work and staying full days. I didn't want to eat in the lunchroom with everyone because I sometimes got the dry heaves when I ate, and I always got the hiccups. So I sat at my computer all day. I did get up every hour and walk around so that I wouldn't impair circulation or anything. After one month, I had lost 50 pounds. I felt good about my decision to have the surgery. I did miss eating a large quantity of food at one sitting. But I can't say my eating time was diminished. I had to take small bites, and then chew and chew. It took a long time to eat. If you don't chew your food very well, it can get stuck, because outlet from your stomach is tiny. It happened to me a couple of times and it was very painful. I just drank small sips of water, and sometimes the food washed through. At other times, I had to make myself throw up. At the end of the second month I had lost a total of 80 pounds. I started walking again, and actually looked in the mirror a few times. I had avoided mirrors like the plague when I was heavy, except to shave in the morning.

The weight kept coming off. My biggest complaint was the gas. I had a lot of really foul gas. My co-workers knew about it and we joked about it. There were times when people got up and left my area because of it. At home, I would actually get up and go outside to pass gas. However, my wife couldn't stand the smell at night and started sleeping in our guest room. She had finally gotten so she could sleep through my snoring—and now this.

After five months I had lost 120 pounds and the gas diminished a little bit. I had an awful taste in my mouth most of the time. It tasted like I had just eaten a tin can. I handled this with constant gum chewing. The funny taste made my food taste bad too. After the fourth month, I didn't notice the taste anymore. After eight months I had lost 185 pounds and was down to 315. I felt better than I had in years. I couldn't wait to cross the 300-pound threshold—which I did in the twelfth month, when I weighed in at 299 pounds. For some reason, that sounded almost normal to me. I know I had never expected to weigh that again. The doctor scheduled me for surgery to get rid of some of the sagging stomach skin. I had that done at the end of the twelfth month. They took off twelve pounds around my stomach and hips. I had to take another week off from work to recover from that surgery. Three months later I weighed 250 pounds and had only 40 pounds to go to get to my high school weight. I really liked how tight and firm my stomach felt.

Over the next six months, the last 30 pounds came off more slowly. When I got to 225, I seemed to stay there for a long time. My doctor said it might be my "set-point" but I did lose a little bit after I started working out at the gym. I decided not to get paranoid about wanting to weigh 210 and I settled for between 220 to 225. I wore size 40 pants and took an extra large shirt, but at least they were off the rack and I no longer had to go to the Big and Tall store. Actually, I had never gone there—my wife did all that for me before, or she had hired a seamstress to make clothes for me. Now I go out shopping for myself. I like to go alone because I spend lots of time looking in the mirror. I never realized I have a passion for clothes, I always wore what fit. But now, I'm starting to notice what colors and styles look good on me. I got my hair redone so it looks wind-blown and rugged and I'm getting quite vain.

The biggest joy has come from rejoining my family mentally and physically. The kids come to me and ask me to play ball or to take them places again. My wife has more time for herself because I'm willing—and able—to help around the house. I can't seem to stop smiling some days because it seems like I was given a new life, and it's better than anything I could have imagined. I can't sit still and watch TV anymore because there is just too much fun stuff to do. I go for a walk or a bike-ride every day because I want to. I still crochet and have made more afghans because it's relaxing and, when I do watch TV, I like to have my hands busy. I no longer worry about dying young, and my blood pressure is normal again. The doctor says I'll live a long and healthy life.

Tammy

I was overweight but didn't really accept that I was. Yes, I wore a size 18 to 20 dress, but I did all the activities a thin person does. When I looked in the mirror, I didn't see myself correctly. I don't know how I did it, but I looked normal to myself, kind of the opposite of anorexia. I thought I was thin, even though I looked quite fat. Actually, from the front I looked okay, it was from the side that I really looked fat. I saw myself from the side in the mirror at the gym and I looked enormous, plus I was beginning to get a double chin. My face had always looked thin with a well-defined chin line and now

I looked fat in the face as well as body. Photographs made me stop and wonder who that fat person was before I realized it was me. I really admired Jack LaLanne who, at 83, had the body of a 29-year year-old. His philosophy was never to eat anything that man has made—white flour, sugar and any processed foods. He also didn't eat meat. I wasn't quite as rigorous as he was, but I tried to eat 10 fruits or vegetables a day, like he did. I didn't try all kinds of diets prior to my gastroplasty, but always tried to eat healthy. I guess I just ate too much, or had a slow metabolism.

I had a whole different experience from stomach surgery because mine was not intentional. I have been slightly overweight since childhood. I was having a great deal of pain in my side as well as unexplained "coffee ground" feces. They were dreadfully black, and very granular. I was concerned, and went into the doctor because of those symptoms. After some tests, which included ultra-sound, a stool culture (yuck) and a sigmoidoscopy (bigger yuck), I was admitted to the hospital for exploratory surgery. The doctors discovered a large grapefruit-sized tumor attached to the gall bladder and extending over to the stomach and small bowel. It was non-malignant but had to be removed. I had had tumors before: thyroid tumor, breast tumors, and one on the ovaries. There are probably others growing in me right now that I don't know about. I seem to be at risk for tumors. My theory is that, when I was a child living in the middle of Colorado during the 1950s, I was exposed to radiation during the testing of atomic bombs that was done in Nevada and southern Utah. The winds were easterly, and the fall-out drifted over where I lived. Of course I have no proof of this, but I do have lots of unexplained tumors, as do others in my town.

The doctors went in to remove the tumor and, with it, my gallbladder, part of my stomach, and five feet of small bowel. As a result of this surgery, I started losing a surprising amount of weight. I was delighted to be dieting without trying. I could no longer eat red meat or fatty foods because of this surgery. The only lingering effect I have is some seepage from my belly button and soreness around the incision.

I also felt full quicker and didn't feel like eating as much because I only had half my stomach. I went from 225 pounds to 150 pounds over the next two years without trying. I'm still active, but now I see the real me when I look in the mirror.

Some minor side effects, like sore hips and a stiff knee, went away completely. I had also experienced some incontinence prior to my surgery. The doctors said the muscles were weak from having six children. They recommended the Kegel exercises, which I did religiously. I think those who promote Kegels must be men, because it didn't make one shred of difference with me. Anyway, it went away after I lost 75 pounds.

Even though I had gastroplasty unintentionally, I would recommend it to anyone. Based on my experience, it can erase some of your health problems and make you feel 20 years younger. My chin-line is back to normal now and my co-workers think I had a face-lift. I am more active than ever before, and now I look the part. I love to go shopping and I've thrown out all my big size clothes. I don't plan on ever being heavy again.

Lacy

I got to the hospital at 6:00 A.M. I was very scared. If I hadn't wanted to die anyway, I would not have gone through with it. I was shaking so badly when the nurse came in that she had to get a heated blanket for me. Then she called in the IV person, and I think they gave me something to calm me down.

I waited on the gurney for about 90 minutes. I was still shaking, and feeling very apprehensive. I didn't really want to go through with this operation, but I felt I had no other choice. I was disgusted with my life. I either wanted it to change or I wanted it to end. The anesthesiologist came in and said they'd had some "complications" with the patient before me. That really did it to my nerves. I wanted to run but, of course, running at 437 pounds is almost impossible.

I wanted to know what the "complications" were with the last patient. The doctor couldn't tell me. I said, "Did she die?" He shook his head but didn't say anything. Then I thought, "Well, what if it was me? At least I'd be through with this miserable life." He told me what was going to happen in the operating room. He told me he'd be monitoring my vital signs carefully, and that nothing was going to happen to me. I asked him if he thought my doctor was up to doing another surgery and he shook his head ever so slightly and said he thought so. That head-shake told me he had been contemplating the same thing.

I was wheeled into the operating room about 11:00 A.M. I looked around at all the instruments, the big light above me and the crash cart. I saw the doctors and nurses all in masks. There was no agreeable banter, no joy at all as far as I could tell. It seemed like they were all absorbed in their own thoughts. I imagined they were thinking about the previous patient. I was glad in a way that I had been told about her, because otherwise everyone's behavior would have seemed sullen. The anesthesiologist started the knock-out stuff in my IV and told me to count backward from 100 by threes. That's a hard task for anyone, but I remember getting to about 88—and then just darkness.

The next thing I knew, I seemed to be standing above my body surrounded by a bright light. There were alarms and beepers going off. The doctors and nurses were frantic. I heard someone yell, "We can't lose two in the same day." Beside each of the doctors and nurses, there seemed to be other people. They were dressed in white and were whispering to them.

Above me were other people dressed in white, who seemed to be standing in a circle with their heads bowed. All the women had veils over their faces. I thought that was very strange. Very Middle-Eastern. I understood that they were praying for me, even though I couldn't hear any words.

I was aware that I had to make a decision. I knew that I needed to decide to go back to my body. I did not want to. I had never felt so free, so alive or so happy. I could move around wherever I wanted by just thinking about it. I had wanted to die, and now I could have my wish if I desired it. However, I also felt that I would be letting my family down if I stayed there. It was with great resignation and astonishment that I decided to go back. At that moment I felt a sucking force bringing me back to my body. It was nothing I could have fought against, because it was so compelling. I felt myself rejoin my body and I felt an excruciating pain for several seconds as that "fusion" happened. It was worse than giving birth. I had never been very religious but, at that moment, decided that maybe religion ought to have some part in my life.

I woke up in recovery at 5:00 P.M. that evening. My first words out were, "I didn't want to come back." The nurse just stared at me. She asked me what I meant. I told her in a croaky voice about the time I had spent out of my body. She confirmed that they thought they had lost me. I was revived after only a few minutes, but she reported that it was considered a miracle because of a blood clot that had traveled to my lungs. She said almost no one survives a clot like that. But she said that it had lifted everyone's spirits to have me come back to the land of the living.

I have lost over 200 pounds. I can finally look in the mirror without avoiding my body when I look. My husband and children seem more precious to me than ever, and I have a zest for life that I never knew before. Part of it is having a new body, and part of it is knowing, without a doubt, that there is life beyond this one. I have begun a new hobby, genealogy. I want to find out who those people were who were praying over me when I had my out of body experience. I am a more religious person than ever before and I am no longer yearning for death. I know that, when it comes, I'll be ready and happy to leave this world behind and go on.

Floyd

My husband, Floyd, decided to have weight loss surgery in the winter of 2002. He had not been feeling well, and his pulmonary consultant decided that he should wait until the spring, because he had a respiratory infection that wouldn't go away. He went into surgery in February of 2003 and everything was fine. He did have to be put on a ventilator for a short time, but it was taken out later. I went home thinking everything was okay. The next day when I walked into the hospital, I found out he had been moved to the surgical intensive care unit and put back on the ventilator.

He was sedated with a drug called Diprivan, which put him to sleep for most of the day. After a week, they said he had to get a feeding tube into his stomach because he wasn't getting enough nourishment through the IV. At this point, he began to get bedsores and severe diarrhea. In addition, he wasn't kept very clean and had anal sores from the diarrhea. He also had the start of sepsis (infection) because of a leak from the surgery. That had to be repaired with more surgery. He spiked a high fever after the second operation and the doctors said it was touch and go for a while. After a month, he was still in the hospital fighting infections, bedsores, diarrhea, and malnutrition. He was able to begin eating baby foods at that point. However, he could only eat about a fourth of a cup before getting overfull. They began to try to roll my husband from side to side using big straps several times a day. If that had been started sooner, perhaps he wouldn't have gotten the bedsores. He couldn't really sit up because of the anal soreness.

The physical therapists told me that they might be able to have him stand up if they rigged up a hoist, so we tried that. The hoist looked like a big harness and was very uncomfortable. However, the physical therapist said it would be the best thing for him, so he tried it several times. The harness took some of the weight off of his feet and he could stand for several minutes before he got real tired and wanted to lie down again.

I could see that things weren't going right and that, if he couldn't even get out of bed on his own, he was a long way from coming home. One of the doctors said he had the bedsores because he was so heavy, and there wasn't anything the hospital could have done about it. I asked him how come he never had them before, even when he was sick and had to stay in bed for a long time at home? He didn't have an answer. In May, we all had a meeting—the doctors, physical therapists and me—to decide how to get him through this and back home. It was decided that he be moved to a rehabilitative care unit where he could be monitored, but allowed to do more things on his own. We moved him to a wonderful facility in June of 2003. By this time the anal sores were under control and he could sit. From there he could stand briefly and transfer weight from foot to foot in preparation for walking.

I was very optimistic at this point and could see the day when he would come home again. He had lost over a hundred pounds of the three hundred he wanted to lose, but was extremely malnourished. My husband told me that he wanted to die, he'd had enough and didn't want to be a burden on me anymore. I couldn't believe what I was hearing. I thought we were getting close to the end but I guess I didn't realize how depressed he was.

About midnight on June 14th 2003, he began to have internal bleeding, and leakage and respiratory distress. The care facility rushed him to the hospital, but the doctor wasn't able to operate until the next morning. By that time they had done a CT scan and determined that he had had a stroke. He was paralyzed and unable to move on his own. They went ahead and operated to control the leakage, but the neurologist said that he would remain in a vegetative state if he lived much longer. It was also hard for him to breathe and he was on a ventilator again. I know that he would not have wanted to live like that, so when the doctors suggested that the ventilator and feeding tubes be withdrawn and he be left to recover or pass away on his own, I knew that was the right thing to do.

I called his family and his mom and dad flew in to say a last good-bye to him. He wasn't responding except with eye movement and groans. He did try to say something to us, but we couldn't make it out. It was probably that he loved us and was sorry.

We disconnected all life support on June 20th, 2003 and my darling husband lived for a few hours and then passed peacefully onto his next journey. I know that we will be together again, and in the next life his body will be perfect. I don't know how much longer he would have lived if he hadn't decided to have weight-loss surgery, but it surely would have been longer than the four months he lived after surgery. But I also know how much he wanted to be thin and to be the kind of man he thought I deserved. I'm not saying anyone is to blame for what happened to my husband, but if I can sway anyone to not have surgery, to just enjoy the life they have, I would. I know I would rather have my husband back the way he was, even at 475 pounds.

Wanda

Good-bye to those cheese fries at Outback Steak House. No more bacon cheeseburgers dripping with mayonnaise. "See ya," five slices of combo pizza with everything on it. "Vamoose" to hidden caches of candy bars that helped me make it through the night. "Adieu" to the pastries I have loved. "So long" cheesecake from Marie Callender. "Adios" to the three chicken fajitas with sour cream I used to die for. "Get out of town" to several helpings of roast pork, beef or chicken at a buffet. "Cheerio" to cake, cookies and pie. "Sayonara" to thick frosty milkshakes. "Depart from me" all you Dove ice cream bars and mile-high mud pie. "See you later," huge meals at Christmas and Thanksgiving.

"Hello" to small quantities of food that would have barely been an appetizer before. "Hi" to loading up on protein shakes that taste like chalky prescriptions. "Salute" to the pills and pills and pills I have to take everyday. "Greetings" to the half glass of juice I can get down in one sitting.

"Salutations" to the quarter apple, the one baby carrot or the tiny cracker it takes me 20 minutes to eat. "Hail" the one-square inch of meat I chew and chew and chew so it won't get stuck in my newly plumbed system and force me to go to the hospital. "Howdy" to the dinner dish no bigger than a hockey puck.

"Hi" to small size clothes at the mall. "Good-bye" to indigestion at night from eating too much. "Hello" to savoring each bite of food instead of scarfing it down without tasting it. "Good-bye" to hurting ankles, legs, back, joints and hips. "Greetings" to adoring glances from my spouse. "Good-bye" to going to bed alone. "Salutations" to athletic activities I never thought I could participate in. "Farewell" to shopping at the big-size clothing store.

The loss of my ability to stuff food in my mouth as fast as I can has been replaced with much more tangible rewards. I love the new me, but mourn the price I had to pay to be this way. I would never go back, and I would do it again tomorrow if I needed to. I would rather be able to eat anything I want to and still look this way, but alas, that was not to be my fate, so I thank my lucky stars that I was born in a time when this alternative is available. My final weight loss was 100 pounds.

I said good-bye to what I thought was important in my life and found out that all that good food really didn't matter very much. I'm glad to be thin, happy to have my family around me, and blessed in the life I'm now living.

Grandma Pat

I am happy to report that I had gastroplasty one year ago and have had nothing but good results. No complications, no depression over not eating my favorite foods, nothing. I have lost over 100 pounds and am a lot happier. For the first time in years my cholesterol is normal (198), and my triglycerides have fallen from 310 to 200. I have gone from 75 units of insulin per day to 10. I think I could get off it entirely if my general practitioner wasn't so skeptical about this change. He's holding on to my old "sick" image, which I have long since discarded. I was 67 years old and I could barely walk when I had the surgery, and I don't know if I had many years left at my former weight. There were so many health risks associated with being overweight and sedentary that I didn't have a chance to live a long and happy life. I had many years of failures on diets before I heard about this "last resort." I wish I would have done it years ago. But in a way I'm happy that I didn't do it before because the results were so unreliable in the past.

You would think that the sagging skin would be a major turn-off for most people, but I can honestly say that I don't think I have more sags than most people my age. I can now do more than I ever did before; it's as if I'd been carrying around a backpack filled with 100 pounds of cargo that I was finally able to put down. I feel light as a feather, and can outlast some of my grand kids at a day in the park.

Some people might think that I was too old to have anything as vain as weight loss surgery. I don't feel as old as the calendar says I am. I did it for my health as well as for my looks, and I've never been more pleased.

Ailene

I am going to have a gastric bypass in the fall. Right now, they are trying to get all my information together in order to present it to my insurance company. I am excited, but also scared stiff. I can't sleep, partly because I have a sleep disorder anyway, but the stress of this is affecting my job and every aspect of my life. And I haven't even done it yet. I keep anticipating all the changes. I'm eating like a hog now because I figure I'll never be able to eat like this again. The doctor showed me a serving spoon when I was in his office. He said, "This is normally what you would use several times to dish up your dinner; after this surgery, your dinner will fit on this spoon."

I can feel myself falling into depression most nights. I wonder if I will still be me. Will I be the same person? I'll have to admit that if some people don't like me afterwards it will no longer be because I'm overweight. I have been rather loudmouthed and abrupt in my demeanor, I think, because I don't want people to think of me as the fat person. So they think of me as that loudmouth. To me, that is better. As I lose weight, will I be able to tone it down a bit or will I still be the loudmouth?

At 55 years of age I've pretty much accepted my physical shortcomings, but the health issues demand I do something. I've tried the diets, and have only ended up fatter and sadder after each one.

I have type II diabetes, hypothyroidism, sleep disorder, and asthma. I weigh 350 pounds, and am over 200 pounds overweight. Most people don't realize how fat I am, I guess, because I'm tall and well proportioned. I also know how to dress to hide all the lumps and bumps. Besides that, I don't think anyone would dare say anything to me about it, and I don't have any real friends.

Part of me says I should accept things as they are and call it off. The other part says I'm being foolish and need to go ahead. I know that if I continue to eat the way I do now—like there is no tomorrow—I will be 300 pounds overweight by the time I get around to the surgery. Then there will be no choice. It will be the surgery, or die within a year. My doctor is already concerned about my blood pressure, which has been as high as 150/110. And recently I've begun to huff and puff going up and down the stairs in my house.

If there were no mirrors to look in, and people accepted me the way I am, I could be happy if I was healthy. But I've faced discrimination from being fat many times over the years. I've gotten overlooked for promotions and overlooked by men. I'm a very nice person inside, but that side can't come out because of how I look. Even my nieces and nephews are afraid of me. I've offered to baby-sit and been turned down, and I know it was the kids themselves. When they were small it didn't matter. But now that they are in school, they see me as a fat person and not as a kind and loving aunt.

There are as many reasons to go ahead with this surgery as there are not to. It's almost as if dying on the hospital gurney would be preferable to going through life as a fat person any longer. I want to see what life holds for me as a thin person. I'm sure it will be different. I only hope it isn't too late to change my mental attitude as my physical image changes.

My doctor is very kind and understanding, but he is as thin as a rail. He's talked to lots of fat women and seen their lives change as they got rid of the weight. He says that the joy this brings him is worth the two negative aspects of his specialty. One is the outrageous insurance costs he has to pay. It isn't always safe to operate on huge people simply because of the wide variety of medical complications that can arise. The other negative is the perspective of other physicians against what he does. In their minds, being overweight is the fault of the person and can be cured by good old-fashioned self-control. They have no idea. I'm sure that one day a discovery will be made that points to a faulty gene, or group of genes, that gives a person the tendency to gain weight disproportionate to the amount of food they consume.

In the meantime, my turn has come. I'm thankful that I can have this surgery and have a chance at a normal life. It's just that I'm scared of the reality of checking into the hospital, putting on the dressing gown, lying down on the table and having the anesthesia go into my veins. I wish I had someone close to me who would help me through it but, like everything else in my life, I have to do it by myself. I may never overcome the fear of going into the hospital alone, but with the passage of time I hope to be grateful that I had the guts to go under the surgeon's knife. I hope everything turns out the way I imagine it will.

Alice

I found out about a doctor in Mexico over the Internet. I didn't do a great deal of research, but I do know that he is fairly-priced, although not the cheapest you can find. He speaks great English, and works out of an excellent facility that is about an 80-minute plane ride south of Houston. I called him directly, and he had his daily planner with him; within a few minutes I had a date for the adjustable gastric band surgery. I chose a date the very next week. It was then up to me to find airline and hotel accommodations. He recommended the Hampton Inn downtown, and so I called. They were able to accommodate me at a reasonable cost of about $90 per night. The trip to Monterrey wasn't bad, with our plane leaving Montana at 11:30 A.M. and arriving at 9:30 P.M., with a two-hour layover in Houston. The doctor had arranged for a van to pick me up from the airport once

I got there. Arriving so late at night, I was deeply grateful for this accommodation.

I checked into the hotel and slept well. Almost all of the employees I dealt with spoke some English. I had wondered about drinking the water, but our hotel had a sign that said the water was purified. I tried it and I didn't have any problem. The next day, the doctor's receptionist called to set up an appointment for 4:30 P.M. At 4:15 P.M. the next day I ordered a taxi and was taken to the clinic, a short distance away. The doctor was late, but when he came in and started explaining things to me, my fears were lessened a great deal. He has had the lap band surgery himself and lost over 90 pounds. That was a great endorsement by itself. How many surgeons have had the same procedure they are about to do to you?

The next day I woke up at 6:00 A.M., and was in the taxi by 6:45. I was taken to the hospital. My taxi driver must have thought it too much trouble to pull up to the door so he let me out on the sidewalk a block away from the hospital. The admittance procedure was very relaxed. A man took my name and address down on a piece of paper and then entered it into a computer. No long forms to fill out, hardly any information at all. I was never given an identification bracelet or anything. I guess it's pretty easy to keep track of the gringos. No one cared about my age or room preference or insurance, or any of the usual things that are pretty standard in the United States.

I was taken to the pre-op area at 7:10 A.M., and the nurse indicated I was to put on a gown. She didn't speak any English. Then I was shown to a bed where I listened to my CD player to calm myself. I was pretty nervous. I have had elective surgery before, and I started wondering the usual.

Waking up once they put me under was the biggest concern. I think it is always a concern when going under anesthesia for any reason. The mistakes are always widely known and we hear about the people who died because of an anesthesia error. It makes the risk loom larger than it probably is. I tried to put other fears out of my mind, and having the music helped.

About 7:30 the anesthesiologist came to talk to me. He spoke perfect English and it was nice to talk to someone who understood me. I told him I was deeply concerned about the tubes going down my throat because after the last surgery I had, I was hoarse for six weeks. I think they damaged the vocal cords. I'm a singer with a church solo coming up within a month—I couldn't afford to have that happen again. He said he'd be very careful. Then he assured me that nothing was going to happen to me and that I would be well taken care of. Then he was off.

While the anesthesiologist was talking, the nurse started the IV. I didn't even feel it so she must have been pretty good. When the doctor was gone, the drip solution had started. For some reason, I've had some pretty bad experiences with nurses starting IV's in the United States because they say I have small veins.

Next, they made me hand over my CD player. I kind of wanted it with me, but I guess that wasn't possible in the operating room. It was hard to ask what they planned to do with it because no one understood me. All communication was done by pantomime and one-word commands. One nurse kept talking to me in Spanish, very loud, as if that would help me to understand her. It didn't.

They wheeled me into the operating room and pointed to the operating table. No one knew how to tell me to "move," so I said "move?" and they nodded. I slid over to the flat operating bed and then the IV was primed with the anesthesia, and that's the last thing I remember until I woke up about 10:30 A.M. in the recovery room. Right in the middle of my abdomen was a tremendous pain. I couldn't communicate with anyone about it and it was a difficult time. Then a doctor who spoke English came by and ordered some pain medication. It didn't help much. He said everything had gone okay and I should be taken to my room within a half an hour.

I really needed my CD player to help distract me. Beautiful music is what helped me get through my labor and delivery many years ago, and I know it would have helped. But no one knew what I wanted because I couldn't speak Spanish.

I was not taken to my room for three hours because it wasn't ready. I also was just left alone for most of the time in my pain because no one could understand me. The doctor had said that I would be given a paper with Spanish phrases on it so that I could at least point to the thing I needed on the paper. However, that paper didn't show up until I was in my room about at 2:00 P.M. At that time I was moaning with pain and the nurse called the doctor and some inter-muscular pain medication was injected. It cut the pain in half, so that it was bearable, but not comfortable. I have a high threshold for pain and I know from previous surgeries that this pain was exceptional. I learned later that the doctor didn't give morphine, and relies on less-effective pain medications. I don't agree with his policy at all. I think that if pain can be controlled, it should be. I'm not going to become a drug addict in one or two days. In the United States, some people are given control over their own pain medication with an apparatus that lets the patient give the medication within controlled parameters. That would have been the only improvement I would suggest to the hospital in Mexico.

Once in my room, I started dangling my legs and standing briefly on my own. No one came in and told me to do it, but I knew that it is good to get up and get going as soon as you possibly can to prevent blood clots and swelling. I had to go to the bathroom as soon as I was shown into my room, but no one understood bathroom, rest room, or toilet. However, when I pantomimed putting a bedpan under me, the nurse said "pee pee?" I nodded and they put a bedpan under me. I went and went and went, a little dribble for about 10 minutes. I don't know why they don't automatically do that every so often when you are given so much IV fluid over a short period of time. I was walking to the bathroom on my own by that night. I tried to unhook the IV myself but not only did it start dripping on the floor, the connection into me began to fill with blood as a vacuum was created. The nurse showed me the proper way to disconnect by turning the flow switch to off.

I was very grateful to the anesthesiologist for inserting the tubes carefully because my voice was fine—I wasn't hoarse at all. My CD player was waiting for me back in my room and I began to sing along with Andrea Bocelli, an octave lower than usual, but there was obviously no damage to my vocal cords.

I began to feel another pain that I hadn't felt before. It was in my left shoulder area and was horrible. However, if I pushed very hard on it, or got up and sat in a chair, or walked around, it would go away briefly. The doctor said later it was a referred pain (originating in another area) from the gas they had pumped into my abdominal cavity during the operation to distend things. He said most patients felt it in their side or back but from my description of how it came and went, he was sure that was the origin of it. He said that pain might be with me for up to a month, off and on. However, it was gone by the next day and never came back.

At one point I asked the nurse—by pointing to the phrase card—to call my doctor because I was in so much pain. Immediately afterwards, an intern appeared who spoke English. I think he was the doctor on call, and he was able to order more pain medication for me.

Later that night, I was given a sleeping/pain pill that was quite effective. I slept well through the night and awoke feeling much better. I was very hungry and was disappointed to see two Jell-O containers and some apple juice for breakfast. It was the same as the dinner I had the night before. The doctor had gotten my hopes up by telling me I would be given a kind of runny cereal made from corn meal that morning and I was looking forward to it. He later admitted he had forgotten to order it. However, the nurses would not consider getting it for me even though I told them the doctor had said I could have it. It was very hard to communicate with them.

I got up, showered and dressed, and waited to be dismissed from the hospital. No one bothered me or came to check on me. However, the previous night, I had noticed that whenever I pushed the nurse button, someone answered within seconds on the intercom. In the United States, my experience with pushing the nurse button is that they come and check on you whenever they darn well please, sometimes it's a half an hour later. I learned to say "dolor" for pain or "baño" if I had to go to the bathroom over the intercom and a nurse would appear within two minutes.

The doctor's assistant came in about 10:00 A.M. to discharge me from the hospital. Their policy is that you have to be out before 11:00 A.M. or else another day's room charge is applied. It was difficult to find out exactly what I had to do to leave but I finally got the taxi to come from the hotel to pick me up and the nurses stopped a random doctor in the hospital so they could communicate with me after I went out to the hallway station and acted like I wanted to leave. He informed me I had to go back into my room to get a final inter-muscular shot for pain before they would let me go.

Finally the taxi came and I walked out to it. No wheelchairs for Mexican hospitals. The nurses waved good-bye. I think they were happy to see me go because it was embarrassing for them and for me to not be able to communicate effectively.

Back at the hotel, I stayed around my room and the pool. I really felt quite good. I had been given some pain pills and I took one about every two hours for minor pain. I slept quite a bit and didn't do much of anything except go out and lie in the sun. The doctor had said I could even go swimming if I felt up to it but I didn't push it. I had their buffet dinner about 8 P.M. I just had soup, but it was delicious and I overdid it, with about two and a half cups. The side pain came back briefly when I got so full. The soup just trickled down to the larger stomach and didn't get hung up in the pouch. At about 10 P.M. the doctor called. He had been out of town for another surgery and wasn't able to get back in time to come and see me. He asked how I was and said he would come by the next day.

The next day he came by the hotel at noon and stayed for about an hour. He is a very personable man and we talked about his family and Mexican culture. I had noticed that Mexicans seemed to be very family-oriented and he agreed. Life there seemed pretty much the same as in the United

States. I went to the mall and had more soup at another buffet. I also had a small roll, but I diluted my mouth with plenty of juice so that it would go down okay and had no problem. I went back to the hotel and sat by the pool. That night I slept very well.

The next morning I was at the airport at 6:00 A.M. for a 7:00 A.M. flight home. The desk clerks at the airport didn't even arrive until 6:30. Some of the people in line were quite worried about the short check-in time before take-off. But I learned that, in Mexico, most deadlines are flexible. I did make my flight in plenty of time and arrived in Houston at 8:30 A.M, and was home about 3:00 P.M. The only complication was some hugely swollen feet from the flight. I should have worn open shoes so my feet wouldn't hurt so much. There were no complications or emergencies for me once home and, in fact, the doctor called again from Mexico. I was happy to report I was fine. I was actually eating most anything by then and didn't notice much of a change at all from having the band put in.

I had hoped to start losing weight immediately, but it was enough just to get used to having the band in place and feeling the food wash through. In the first month I barely lost 10 pounds, and that was by going on Weight Watchers. I didn't think I would ever have to diet again, but I certainly wasn't going to go through with this surgery and then gain weight the first month. My insides felt slightly bruised when I ate, but not too bad. I did have to drink more water than normal with every bite or things got stuck. When food got stuck it was painful, and felt like heartburn. I got hung up on a roll (eaten without water to mush it up), a carrot, and some meat. I guess the weight loss starts after the first adjustment (or fill) is made after four weeks and the opening from the pouch to the larger stomach area is tightened. In a way, I'm not looking forward to that. I think this will be weight loss through pain, judging by the way I feel whenever food gets hung up in the pouch and won't go through right away. It backs up into my throat and doesn't feel very good until I burp or the wave action of the stomach washes it down—I usually get hiccups with each meal. It's a different way to eat, that's for sure. I hadn't expected it to be painful to eat. To avoid the pain I drank with each bite so that the food would go through the aperture. However, that defeats the purpose of the band.

I feel like I accomplished a victory just by going to Mexico by myself and braving the different obstacles that were put in my way. After one year I had lost only 20 pounds. I had one "fill" to close down the band, but it was so uncomfortable to eat that I didn't go back for more. I guess I'm one of the people who the adjustable band doesn't work for. I wish I had looked into other options before deciding on the band.

Beverly

I had an adjustable gastric band operation in December of 1999. I was not prepared for the consequences. The things that I thought I knew were: I would lose weight without effort and would have to eat smaller portions. What I didn't know: once the band is in, it is fully expanded, and the opening from your new gastric pouch to the larger stomach is a little larger than half an inch. This does not have much of an effect on appetite, eating patterns or weight loss.

With the band in, I started out on a liquid diet. The second day after the surgery I ate about two cups of clear broth at dinner. I would never have eaten that much soup normally, but it was all I thought I could have. I gradually learned by experimentation that I could eat anything I wanted without consequence if I just diluted it a lot with water as I ate. So my eating pattern became: take a bite, drink some water, repeat. The water would help wash the food down and I could actually feel it going through the band. Sometimes I would burp as the food went into the lower portion of my stomach with a plop. I almost never got blocked, or felt full with a tiny bit of food, as I had expected I would. I felt blocked three times: once with a sandwich that I hadn't drunk any water with. Another time it was with some rice, and once more with celery. I was driving when I ate a stalk of celery. I could feel the back up. It impaired my ability to operate the car as I felt the urge to throw-up and gagged and heaved a few times before I was able to stop. I finally stopped the car and got out. The food came up as I leaned over and I felt much better.

The thing that wasn't discussed with me ahead of time is how painful it is when the system is blocked. It feels like extended heartburn. It is as if an iron hot poker is burning in your stomach. I felt like throwing up all three times the system backed up, but only the celery came up. I had drunk a fair amount of water with the celery, but the texture was such that the chunks formed a block. However, when I leaned over, it ran out of my mouth. It wasn't so much throwing up as gravity.

The sandwich that I ate was very painful. I kept drinking water afterwards, but I could feel that the contents of my esophagus were backing up in my throat. The water wouldn't mix with the texture of the roll, and it was half an hour until the normal wave action of my stomach eventually got the food through. I felt like a clogged toilet that kept filling with water but wouldn't go down.

I didn't lose a lot of weight the first month. In fact, the seven or eight pounds I did lose was during the first week. After that, I could pretty much eat as I had before. My doctor suggested going on a diet. I thought I was done with diets for good. Here I had paid a lot of money for a procedure I now didn't believe in because I was told I would never have to *diet* again. The Atkins diet was suggested. However, I felt so lethargic on it that I chose the Weight Watchers diet instead. One thing that would have pushed me over the edge would have been to gain weight after having gone through so much trouble and pain.

Then, after four weeks, they did the first "adjustment," or "fill," as they call it. This is where the doctor finds the port—which is just under the skin of the breastbone in my case—then injects about 2 ccs of sterile water into the inner-tube portion of the band. This filled it up slightly, and the opening from pouch to stomach was now only about three-eighths of an inch. This had an immediate affect on my ability to eat. I now had to eat very small portions and chew them well or the opening got blocked. The blockage is excruciatingly painful. That is a fact no one mentioned to me prior to surgery. It's weight loss by suffering. You become adversely conditioned to food. Food is now the enemy because it causes agony. Hunger isn't as bad as the pain of eating. Every bite must be well chewed and diluted with plenty of water to ensure that it will get through. The doctor recommends you not drink any water with your meals, but doing it that way, I could only eat a couple of spoonfuls before I felt my esophagus was backing up with food, which was horribly painful. I guess that was the point, but I just couldn't go through it with every meal.

It was especially bad at work, where I might bend over to

pick something up and have food spill out of my mouth after eating. I had this happen so much that I finally refused to eat anything at all at work.

That's when the weight loss starts. I was sorely tempted to have the water removed from my band, and just stay fat. The punishment of eating after having the "fill" didn't seem worth the weight loss. And to think that my body will eventually adjust to meals of this size, and I'll eventually have to eat this way or risk gaining back huge amounts of weight. I'm feeling very sorry for myself. Sorry that I couldn't lose weight without this surgery and sorry I had this procedure in the first place. It was a no-win situation. When people tell me I look great, I say, "Yeah, but I feel like hell." Then I tell them what I did to my body.

The other thing that wasn't mentioned to me before I had the surgery was that constipation is constant with the gastric band. I finally found the solution to that problem with Metamucil wafers and/or liquid. I had to have some everyday to even approach a normal bowel function. Some people get diarrhea, but it was the opposite for me.

Any time the body is altered there will be problems. I can only eat a few hundred calories a day, and feel like I'm starving to death each and every day. The first three letters of diet are die, and that is what I feel like doing.

I now understand why so many patients were there for "revisions," as I noticed in my doctor's waiting room. I think they wanted to be re-plumbed, and have the gastric bypass instead of the restrictive operation so that they could at least eat something. With the bypass operations, what you do eat is not digested properly or fully, and much of it passes from your body without doing any good, or harm (weight-gain). There is a higher percentage of weight loss with the bypass operations, but you have to eat small portions. There are also the side effects—gas, bad breath, abdominal distress, the Dumping Syndrome—and you have to avoid any sugar. All this just to be thin. Is it really worth it?

If I had a suggestion to give to anyone considering this procedure, it would be to be prepared for the worst, and then some. The outcome of weight loss does not balance out the anguish, the expense, the embarrassment when uncontrolled things happen when you eat (like burping or spitting up) or the sorrow at having to give up one of the few pleasures in your life: eating. This wasn't the answer for me, and I haven't lost much weight at all, just 30 pounds in six months.

Tex

Hi! My name is Tex. I had my surgery done in Arkansas, and they do it a little bit differently in the clinic I went to. I had what I thought would be a more moderate approach to surgery. Instead of making a little stomach pouch the size of a golf ball that emptied into the larger stomach, my surgeon decided to use a larger pouch. In fact, it is almost one-half of the original stomach size. Then the Marlex band opening that is supposed to hold back the food for a while was made smaller, so that the food would go through more slowly. I think it is about one-quarter inch in diameter. I thought this would be great because I could eat more food at one sitting, but only one-half of what I used to eat. This would eliminate the vomiting and uncomfortable constrictions that occur when overeating with the small pouch. I had seen my wife struggle with overeating with the regular small pouch. She would get so sick that her face would turn white and she would hold her chest and say she felt like she was having a heart attack. The only relief was if she made herself throw up some of what she had eaten so that it wouldn't back up into the esophagus and make her feel horrible.

There are side effects with any choice we make and, unbeknownst to me, the result of having this half-stomach and smaller outlet was that the food sits for a long time before moving on. I do feel full most of the time. However, I've decided that because the food must sit so long in the stomach acid and saliva, it starts to decompose or rot or something. Consequently I have a very bad taste in my mouth most of the time. It tastes somewhat like my household garbage can smells. And my wife and others report that my breath could kill. I have started trying to get the food to go through faster by drinking lots and lots of water with meals and chewing until the food is the consistency of baby food. Sometimes that works, but then I'm still hungry because my saturation point hasn't been reached. And it's still difficult to get meats and vegetables to go through very fast because of the texture of those foods. Sometimes I take my meat and put it in the blender with the vegetables and eat it like mush. I still have to drink excess water to get it to go through the band. I can imagine the rest of my life will be like this, and I'll just start shopping in the baby food aisle for my meals.

It's been a bother as far as eating. The pleasure of eating has gone. It is now a chore to plan and execute how I am going to eat a food and how I can get it to go through the opening faster. I may have to go in for a revision of the procedure at some point. However, insurance won't pay for it, and it will be in excess of $15,000. So I will have to wait. The doctor won't arrange for payments—he wants to be paid before the surgery begins.

As·for my weight, that too has been a disappointment. I lost about ten pounds the first week, and then ten more pounds over the next two months, and then I stopped losing anything. It's rather sad, because I had all these plans to throw out my old, larger clothes and get a new wardrobe. I still go shopping and buy the same size. It does fit a little better than it did twenty pounds ago, but it's the same size I was. I feel so defeated to think I may have to go on another diet. I have re-joined Weight Watchers over forty times in my life, and to do it again, after having this surgery, just seems very unfair to me. Vomiting is the worst, because of the length of time food sits in my stomach. It tastes like acid when it comes up but, sometimes, the only way I make it through the day is to throw up what I eat. I can't lose weight, I can't afford a take-down, I can't afford a revision, and I have huge consequences that I hate minute by minute.

I can only hope that I can keep the weight off a little bit better with this smaller stomach. And maybe my sense of smell will diminish as I age, so the garbage taste in my mouth will go away, or maybe I'll just get used to it. I may never be allowed to kiss my wife again because of her revulsion, but I can chew breath gum all day when I go to work.

For me, it hasn't worked out the way I had hoped, but there are still things that can be done, like opening the Marlex band to about a half an inch. I think that would take care of the lingering smell and mouth taste. I may even have the stomach banded higher up, so that I will eat less. That will be a couple of years down the road, when we have enough money. I'm not looking forward to it, but I still have hope that I'll eventually be thin. I wish I had talked to another person who had gone through this ordeal before I went ahead and agreed to my doctor's plan. It sounded good the way he explained it, but he left out some important details, like the taste in my mouth and the breath smell.

Keith

I had an unusual consequence from my adjustable gastric band surgery that was done on the 11th of March, 2002. I had been bulimic for my whole adult life—about 30 years. I had managed to control it at times; there was even a two-year period when I wasn't bothered by it at all. However, repeated counseling, pills and doctors had not cured the problem. That is, until I had the band put in. Then I was unable to throw up in my usual fashion. I tried several times, but food would not pass up and out from the lower stomach. The result was just a painful stomachache, and me wondering if I had undone the gastric band.

Nowadays, I will overeat for the size of my stomach, which might be a small meal like a half a potato and half a pork chop with some peas. Then I'll get a painful bloated feeling in my esophagus until I throw up the food that is blocking the opening. This is not food that had already gone down into the larger stomach. It is food that is just sitting there in the small pouch, blocking the opening and feeling like hell. I will spit up several bites of food, and they come up in bites. This isn't the quarts and gallons of liquid food I had thrown up when truly bulimic.

When I was bulimic, I had uncontrollable urges to eat thousands of calories at a time—whole cakes, batches of cookies, or several muffins or doughnuts at a time—only to empty out my stomach by throwing up, and then doing it all over again. I had to be careful at the office to hide my eating. I went into the single unisex bathroom on another floor because, on our floor, we had several urinals and two rather public stalls (not sound-proof). I could eat in the stalls, but not throw up, because someone might come in. For some reason, I seem to have a need to do something hidden and covert in my life, because I turned to something even worse when I could no longer practice bulimia.

Bulimia must have been filling a need for me that was essential to my well-being. When I was forced to stop because of the surgery, you would think I would have been happy, because it had been an ugly secret for so long. Though I was intellectually happy, emotionally, I was a wreck. I needed the relaxation and release that eating until stuffed, and then relieving myself, provided. Without that release, my emotional side looked for another way to handle stress. Before, I had always stuffed feelings inside—eating was another metaphor for stuffing myself and my feelings. I suddenly could not do that. I frantically tried exercising, but I found it didn't do the same thing for me. I could exercise on the treadmill or stationary bike for an hour and still feel all anxious and confused inside.

When I was younger, I had a problem with shoplifting. I think that most of the shoplifters are young, or women, because the stores don't seem to look very hard at me. I guess it is unusual to have a man enjoy shopping like I do. I had pretty well overcome the tendency to steal, and did not stuff my booster bags with contraband and sneak out of the store any longer, before the surgery.

However, when the pressure of life built up inside me and I no longer had the luxury of overeating to the point of pain and then getting rid of the pain and guilt by throwing up, I found myself taking things from stores again. I was really puzzled as to why I was doing it. I didn't need to, financially. We were doing okay, and I could buy whatever I wanted within reason. My wife never asked me to account for my money. So I wondered, why I was revisiting this dangerous pastime? I recognized that, sooner or later, I would be caught. I had been caught twice before when I was much younger, and I knew how embarrassing it was. Going before the judge, paying the criminal and civil fines, wasn't worth it. I was blatant enough to just pick up a pair of shoes in Nordstrom and walk out with them right in my hand, not even hidden or anything, and not checking around for store personnel. Why would I do that? It was almost like I wanted to get caught. I loaded a grocery basket with sports equipment at a larger store chain and then, after buying groceries, just wheeled the loaded cart out of the store with my groceries like I had paid for everything. In fact, a clerk came and helped me because she thought I couldn't handle two carts. I happily let her. I guess she thought that, since one cart had sacks of stuff in it that had obviously been paid for, the sports stuff was too big to put into bags, and so it was just put into the cart as is. That got me about $500 worth of stuff that I didn't really want or need. Other days were the same, and I was stealing huge quantities of goods I didn't want or need for some unknown reason. The fact that I used to eat huge quantities of food that I didn't want or need didn't escape my notice. There was some relationship there, but I didn't know what it was. My clothes closet was filing up with clothes, many of which still had the tags on. My wife was also getting an unusual number of gifts from me. Sometimes, when she wanted to take something back for another size or item, she would ask for the receipt. I could never seem to find it, so she had to take things back without one. But she never questioned me about the sudden shopping sprees. She probably

figured I was overdoing shopping so that I wouldn't be thinking about food anymore.

Continuing to get away with shoplifting only fueled my
unmet needs for attention and risk-taking. The rush I get
from getting away with the goods is like an addiction. My face
gets flushed and my heart rate goes up. I recognize that both
things also happened during bulimic purging. I think that,
like a balloon with a weak side, my life had to bulge out
somewhere to relieve the pressure that was building. My normal relief valve was bulimia. Now that an adjustable gastric
band artificially controlled my purging, I couldn't eat anything I wanted as fast as I wanted. With the band in place
those kinds of behaviors led to immediate and instantaneous
agony. So another "bad" part of me reemerged from the
shadows where it had been hiding all these years.

Sometimes, when I'm standing in the bathroom with
overwhelming pain because of overeating a few mouthfuls, I
wish I had never had the band put in. Being fat wasn't pretty or healthy, nor was eating and throwing up several times a
week. But they were the vices and methods of coping that I
had come up with that seemed to work for me. With those
options gone, I turned to stealing to get my jollies. Risk and
the possibility of discovery, possible embarrassment and
shame, seemed to be important to both sets of behaviors.
Also, bulimia has to do with eating lots of food, and shoplifting has to do with getting lots of stuff. Maybe I just feel
deprived and I will do anything to make that feeling go away.
I hope I don't graduate to banks or something, because I
really don't want to end up in jail.

I don't know if I have a behavior problem or a personality disorder or what, but the surgery resulted in a compulsive
tendency of mine that I consider worse than bulimia. I don't

know what to do with myself, because this is not the person I want to be. For me, having the band put in made my life worse than it was before, because it took away something disgusting and replaced it with something shocking and potentially life-ruining. Yes, I lost 100 pounds of fat, but replaced it with a ton of guilt.

Phyllis

I am one of those people who is less than delighted with the results of my vertical banded gastroplasty. I have always been fat, and always wanted to be thin. I remember my first diet was when I was in grade school. My mother sent me to many physicians, and I was on countless diets and pills to no avail. One doctor told me my breath stunk and asked why didn't I just drink water if I was hungry? I was hungry all the time. Instead of accepting myself the way I was, I kept trying more and more diets, pills, and techniques, and wasted lots of time trying to be someone I wasn't. The subtle pressure of mom and dad didn't help me. Dad would bargain, "If you lose this much weight, I'll buy you this or that." Mom would only take me shopping at the thrift store or make my clothes. There really wasn't much available at that time for big kids.

I was bound and determined to go through with this surgery because I saw it as my last chance to be thin. But now I wish I hadn't done it, and I'm not sure I could have been convinced, back when I was thinking about it. What would it have taken to convince me not to go through with the surgery? Probably nothing could have, because I'm pretty stubborn, and I was so sure this was the answer for me at last.

My husband went with me to the first meeting that was held in my city. He was not very supportive, but I suspected it was because of the hefty expense involved. He said he loved me as I was. I felt good when he said that. If he had kept it up and convinced me that he was really happy with me the way I was, I think I might have been persuaded to forego the surgery. But he also would have had to start treating me differently, being more attentive and appreciative. I think some guys actually do like the way a big woman feels, soft and feminine. But how that translates into how she looks in clothes, or how she looks hanging on his arm, is something else again. If my husband had kept assuring me by words and actions that he appreciated my size, I would have been more content with the status quo.

When we got to the meeting, my husband changed his view entirely. He learned that insurance often paid for this procedure, and he was suddenly all for it. Then when he saw the pictures that they passed around of women just like me before and after surgery, he was 100 percent behind me having the surgery. He wanted me to look good, and that meant being thin. That attitude mirrored my own, so I went ahead with the surgery. I was dreadfully afraid of the procedure and didn't want to spend the money, which came from our retirement fund, but I was convinced that it would be worth the risk and the discomfort, and the expense.

I had some serious complications in the hospital. One was something like *ileus*. when your whole GI system shuts down. I had to have stomach tubes and a pickline in my IV (huge hole), and anchors in my insides to hold things together. It took four weeks to even get out of the hospital.

After six months I had only lost 20 pounds. The reason is that it's so easy to get sweets to pass through the restricted opening into my stomach. I've always loved desserts, and the candy melts en route, the cake and cookies get dissolved with the milk I drink, and the ice cream just floats on through. When I get a blockage, it is with something like rice, pasta or red meat. These are things I only eat at dinner, and not for snacks. Then the blockage is very painful for at least 30 minutes. I'm still hungry, my food is still waiting for me, but I have to get up and walk around a bit, or bounce around to get the food to pass through the little hole with a burp. The whole time it feels like colossal heartburn, and I am in agony. My mouth waters uncontrollably, I cry, my jaw and shoulders hurt, and I sometimes wonder what the difference is between this and a heart attack. It feels like those detestable gigantic hiccups that are so difficult to suppress, and are painful besides. Sometimes I try to throw up the little bit of food I ate. When it comes up, the unpleasant feeling goes away a lot sooner. When my band closes up on me I have to get scoped out, and my undigested rotten food is pushed through the pouch into my regular stomach. I don't feel healthy or happy. I wish celebrities like Carnie Wilson would stay out of it. She never shows both sides of her surgery. I hate all the advertising nowadays. No doubt, the weight loss surgeons are paying these people. What a racket they have going.

It's embarrassing to start to burp and hiccup at dinner. It's no fun to have to go walk around while others are finishing their meal in peace. If I'm alone, I kind of jump in place, trying to get the food to go down.

I guess if I had a suggestion for others, it would be to examine their lifestyle rather minutely before going ahead with the surgery. If you love to snack on high-sugar and high-fat foods, it will be easy for you to bypass the control that you are artificially putting into your body in the shape of narrow restrictive bands, because there are tricks to eating all the high-fat and sugary foods you want. You can drink shakes, or eat smaller bites with huge amounts of water, to help wash food through the restriction. The other re-plumbing procedure, where some of the small intestine is bypassed, will be better for you, because you are not allowed to eat sweets with that procedure. Also, some of what you eat is not absorbed properly because of the missing small intestine. Even if someone told me I couldn't eat sweets, I'm afraid that, with my personality, I would just go ahead and eat them all the more and then suffer the consequences.

I guess I could go back and have a revision done and have the bypass put in place but, at this point, I just want to get on with my life and try to live as fully as I can with the body I have. I read that the average female in America wears a size 16 dress. I'm not too far away from that. Recently I got a massage, and the young woman who gave me the massage told me my body was perfect. I have never heard that before in any connection with my body. Oh, for more of that attitude in the world! If I could believe it, I would truly be a happier person.

Deedee

I heard about surgical solutions for weight loss on TV; they are widely advertised where I live. I called the clinic, and they had me come to one of two regularly scheduled get-acquainted lectures that they have each week. There were about 50 people there. Most of them were moderately to severely obese. The good points of the surgery were mentioned, and testimonials were given by those who had undergone one of the procedures. Most of them seemed to work in the office of the doctor. Also, huge numbers of pills, up to 48 per day, and supplemental drinks, were shown to us. This is what they need to take every day to stay healthy after surgery. All of those things require a continual outlay of cash, in addition to the $15,000 to $20,000 cost of the surgery itself.

Everyone was invited to have the doctor put his hand around their wrist at the end of the program, so that he could tell you what size frame you had and what dress size you should eventually have after the surgery. I'd always been told I had a big frame because my wrist measures 7 inches. He told me I'd be a 9–10. I have never been that small; even in junior high I wore a size 12–14.

It was all too good to be true. As with other things that seem too good to be true, I was hesitant. I began researching the surgery and talking to people who had it, or who knew of people who did.

What I found out was that the surgery does work. Most of the people had lost a huge amount of weight, from 50 to 100 pounds or more. But they were miserable. One of the joys of life, eating, was gone. Instead of being able to enjoy food, they now had to eat tiny amounts at a time. They suffered from digestive problems, uncontrolled diarrhea and gas, and they all shared feelings of deprivation. Being in front of a piece of pie, and not being physically able to eat more than a couple of tablespoons, was like putting a starving person in front of a feast and then sewing his lips together.

If they did eat more than they should, it resulted in gastronomic pain so severe that they had to self-induce vomiting—if it didn't happen automatically—to clear the blocked feeling out of their gut. Half the time they felt deprived and, the other half, uncomfortable. Someone described feeling, "Like I swallowed a golf ball." I remember someone saying that lots of long-term complications have yet to be proved, but that kidney stones, hernias, lupus, and autoimmune problems develop after surgery. When I searched on the Internet, I found and astounding number of long-term problems associated with weight loss surgery. Some said that, after a few years, the body adjusted so much that they again had to go on a diet to maintain their weight, but now they could only eat 500 calories a day without regaining weight.

I eventually decided not to go ahead with the surgery, although it is always in the back of my mind. I'm just too satisfied with myself as I am, even though other people consider me fat. If I don't think about it, I just consider myself normal. If only there weren't any mirrors.

Boris

I've always been driven, and achievement-oriented. The fact that I couldn't control my weight had been the thorn in my side since as early as I can remember. My parents died in an auto accident when I was young. They were the most wonderful people on the face of the earth. I think that, psychologically, I have felt I had to live life for them—to get from life what they were denied. And a part of me has always wondered why wasn't I with them in the car that day? Why didn't I die with them?

From the time when I was a child, I always wanted to make things better—I would rearrange reality to make it more bearable. Rather than saying that my parents were dead, I used to tell my friends that they were Hollywood actors who wanted to protect me from the publicity, and so I had to live with my grandma under an assumed name.

However, my teachers and friends didn't quite know how to deal with me. They called me a liar. But I didn't consider it lying—just rearranging the facts to make a bad situation tolerable.

I lied to myself as well. I pretended I was just "healthy," but not fat. I did all the things I wanted to do and never let my weight hold me back. I made sure there were no pictures of me below chest height. It was hard to lie to the doctors. I wouldn't get on their scales, but told the nurses what I weighed instead. I made up the story that, if I saw my weight, my blood pressure would go up and they wouldn't get a good reading. However, when I started to have physical symptoms that were definitely a result of my weight, I had to admit to myself that I was too heavy.

When I reached 400 pounds, I could no longer cover up in a well-cut suit. I walked like a duck because of my fat thighs and knees. My hips, knees, and ankles hurt more than I could bear, but I couldn't lose weight and keep it off. Every day I would wake up and say to myself that today I would be in control. Today I would eat a small amount and exercise and start a healthy life-style. However, it never happened. Around three or four in the afternoon I would start with a trip to the candy machine. Then I would get a snack to sustain me for the long commute home. From then until bedtime I would eat nonstop, until I fell into a blissful coma-like sleep and awoke the next morning not even hungry, and filled with resolve to eat sensibly. It was almost like being an alcoholic who promises himself to be sober in the morning and falls off the wagon by 3 P.M.

I think that wanting to have weight loss surgery was just another lie I told myself. It was a way to be thin without having to take responsibility for my actions. I could allow someone else to perform a procedure on me that would result in weight loss without much being expected of me.

I chose the medial re-section of my bowel because I was afraid that with a distal re-section I would have too much gas.

There wasn't much to the surgery and it was like any other elective surgery. You go in like a frightened puppy, and come out of anesthesia hurting and wondering why on earth you went through with it. But the recovery wasn't unusually difficult or anything. I was back to work within two weeks, after having lost a great deal of weight—twenty pounds in two weeks. But then I got hungry. It was like the whole attention of my conscious mind was focused on food and what I couldn't have. I could no longer have sugar of any kind, except in fruit and vegetables. Table sugar caused a horribly ugly reaction that is so painful that it should proscribe ever eating sugar again, it is so bad!

After two weeks I decided to test the Dumping Syndrome, by having a strawberry shake from Dairy Queen. The glorious taste and texture were awesome. I had missed the exhilarating joy of being pleasantly transported by a tasty treat. My joy was short-lived however as the drink made its way rapidly out of my small stomach pouch and into the new mixing place in my gut. This is the place where the food I eat and the gastric juices from my re-sected larger stomach and gut now meet and begin digestion. I was driving the car at the time. Had I not been at a stoplight when the attack hit, I would have caused an accident. As it was, I couldn't drive farther, but sat in my car feeling kind of glazed and sickened. My face flushed, my heart started racing and I was nauseous to the point that I thought I would throw up at any moment. My body went into dry heaves, but the shake wouldn't come back up—it was too far along in my system.

I started to breathe heavily, and thought briefly that I was having a heart attack. The pain in my gut was overwhelming. In fact, other drivers called 911 for me and an aid car arrived. The paramedic took one look at me and called for an ambulance to take me to the hospital. Vital signs were horrific. My blood pressure was sky-high. He quoted the numbers of 240 over 140. I think that is almost synonymous with death. But within about 20 minutes the symptoms had started to abate.

By the time the ambulance got there, I was breathing normally, my color had returned and was now only kind of ashen. My blood pressure had gone down and my heart was back near normal. I told them what had occurred, but no one had ever heard of the Dumping Syndrome, and I was driven to the hospital anyway for a checkup.

I was released within an hour with the medical staff scratching their heads and wondering why I had even been brought in. I think I educated them that day about the dumping syndrome.

You would think that I would be cured, that the one time I ate sugar and had such a repulsive reaction would have taught me a lesson. But my longing for sweets only got worse. I then started playing a game of Russian roulette with myself. I would buy some chocolate, a brownie, some cookies or something equally filled with sugar and then wait until bedtime to eat it, knowing what was to come. The reaction was always the same. The horrible brush with death would occur, but the five to ten minutes that I had before the reaction, while my mouth and stomach were filling with the delectable, luscious, heavenly taste, was worth the reaction even though it was always as bad as it had been the first time in the car. The only difference was that now I knew what to expect, and how long it would last.

One of these days I may not wake up from these episodes. I can't seem to control myself. A comparison to a drug addict comes to mind. Wanting the rush that drugs bring only, in this case, the taste of food—specifically sweets—is the driving factor. I've lost over 100 pounds but, probably because of my addiction to sweets, I have reached a plateau and don't seem to be losing anymore.

I have passed over the other ramifications of the procedure because I wanted to describe the reaction I have each and every time I eat sweets. After two years, I still test the Dumping Syndrome almost daily, and I've had two hernias and three rope adhesions that gave me a lot of abdominal pain. Of course it was more surgery to fix all of that. It is abhorrent to me to be sitting in front of a nice meal and to be able to eat only a few mouthfuls. I don't get "full" as they said I would, not even close. I am ravenous. But I can't eat more than about one-fourth of a cup at one time. Eating is something equal to a consecrated, holy act for me, and to be denied food is another way to go through hell. My doctor said that some people only have the Dumping Syndrome for a few years and then it goes away. I truly hope I am one of those people.

The pain in my knees and hips has gotten better. I look okay in a well-tailored suit. At 295 pounds I can even get dates, and I feel better about how I look. But a big part of my life is missing. I think that eating sweets, despite the consequences, is proof enough of that. I feel emptier inside than I ever have before, and dying doesn't seem like too big a price to pay, because I hate my life as it is now. No rearranging of the truth in my mind can ever make this situation positive. I am now saving up to have my surgery reversed. It is a hard decision, not only because of the food issue. I am dealing with the horrible Dumping Syndrome almost daily. But the physical effects on my knees and hips will undoubtedly return. I have decided that I would rather eat the way I did before than anything else, even if I have to be obese and have physical distress because of it.

My life is a mess at present and suicide isn't out of the realm of possibility. I believe in the afterlife, and want to see Mom and Dad again. I think, in a way, my acceptance of the dumping syndrome in my life and its consequent reactions are ways that I am trying to kill myself without actually pulling the trigger. It's a catch–22: If I regain the weight, I may die from physical consequences and, if I continue to binge on sweets and suffer the consequences of that, I may die. I wish I would never have heard about weight loss surgery and had taken more responsibility for my eating and exercise program. But I wanted to have my cake and eat it too, both figuratively and literally.

Kiki

I have a complaint about weight loss surgery and that is that the doctors are all nice when they're trying to hook you in. Then you have the surgery and it's like they don't want anything more to do with you. I had the bileopancreatic diversion and then had some major complications. My insurance didn't cover the original surgery, so of course it wouldn't cover any of the costs of the complications.

I would think that the bariatric doctor might help you through some of the downside on the other end, but mine just wanted to hand me off to someone else. It was like I was no longer his problem, even though they had created big problems in my gut. I had such bad contraction-like pains and gas after my surgery, that I could hardly walk. This continued without abatement for about two months, while I mostly stayed in bed wearing a diaper and with a heating pad on my stomach for relief. Yes, I lost tons of weight, but I hardly ate anything because it came out almost as whole food at the other end. During that time, I tried and tried to get my surgeon to do something. He told me to go to my family doctor and get a referral to a urologist. I had fecal incontinence, and if you don't think that impaired my life, think again. I couldn't even leave the house. I had to declare disability and quit my job. I was on the reduced pay they give at my office, and then had horrendous bills associated with trying to get some relief from the pain and incontinence I was experiencing. We've been taught not to poop in our pants since we were little, and now I have no control over it.

Normally, my insurance would have paid to have an operation to lessen the constant draining from my bowels but, since the problem had started after the other surgery and was, in effect, a result of it, the company wouldn't touch it. Now, after going $20,000 in debt and having to declare bankruptcy, I have some control over my bowels. It's not like it used to be, and I still have to wear an adult diaper, but at least I can leave the house. When you have bladder leakage, it is bearable because, if you have an accident, it isn't smelly. However, if you are in public and have a fecal accident, the whole world knows about it because of the smell. With a baby it's kind of cute, but with an adult, you are shunned by strangers, friends, and family. The smell gets to them, and to me too, but I have to live with myself.

I can't believe I did this. Why didn't someone warn me ahead of time about the horrible possibilities? I only heard the positive side from the ladies the doctor recruited to give a presentation to a bunch of people. I would tell anyone that was considering having the surgery to first ask other people who have been to your doctor to describe their experiences. All bariatric surgeons can't be as mean as mine was afterwards.

Before the surgery he had me eating out of his hand. I think I would have done anything he said. He was holding out the Holy Grail. He dropped me like a hot potato, and wouldn't even schedule a follow-up appointment when he found out how big my problems were. The future for me is grim—maybe a colostomy (a bag for my bowel movements) but, since most of my stomach was removed, it can't be reversed. Without any money, or any means of getting any money, there aren't any doctors jumping in line to take my case.

I used to go to the support groups, but it was just too embarrassing, and you would think those people would understand. As an aside, about four people from our support group died during the years I went. I miss those people, and think anyone considering surgery should go to at least two to three support groups before they have the procedure. They won't just be told the sugar-coated side of weight loss surgery.

Sal and Sandy

My wife and I decided to have this procedure done together. We were both overweight and tired of it. I didn't want to see my wife getting thin without me, and she didn't want me to get thin without her. We wanted to go through the changes, whatever they were, together.

I don't think that describing the operation and its ensuing effects is an adequate way to encourage or discourage anyone to go ahead with it. But I am still ambivalent about the results. On the one hand, I look great and so does my wife. On the other hand, we both feel lousy most of the time. Not physically—most of our health problems have gone away. The stiffness, the aches, the backaches are things of the past. However, I still have about 10 to 15 bowel movements a day, and my gas smells like a barnyard. I also lost half my hair and have adult acne. I never even had adolescent acne. My feelings about eating are all negative. Food is no longer a joy to look forward to, but has become a drudgery. It is hard to eat now. That's weird to say, because eating is not usually a hard thing to do; if you can get your hand to your mouth, it's usually fairly straightforward. Now, however, we have to chew and chew small bites. Then, after one-fourth a cup of food, we can't eat any more. Not because we don't want to, we want to very much. But we know that if we do, the consequences and pain in the gut are overwhelming. So we wait for the food to wash down into the stomach, and then eat a little tiny bit more. A meal that used to take 15 minutes to consume now takes over two hours, because we have to wait to eat more. Plus, we never feel really satisfied. It's like deprivation, with a feast in front of us. I lost 50 pounds, and my wife lost 100, but it wasn't worth it. I get checked for malnutrition every three months, and something is always low. My skin is pasty, and my wife just doesn't look as vibrant as she used to, even though she was fatter. We've made our healthy digestive track unhealthy, and just don't feel very good anymore.

As older people, we were okay with the way we looked. There came a point in our lives where we no longer had to be skinny to please the rest of the world. We just wanted to be able to do the things our other skinny friends did, instead of always sitting at home and watching TV. Now, however, we sit at home and try to eat a little at a time, then drink the four protein shakes a day and take handfuls of pills every two hours. Before having the procedure, I was constantly thinking about food, what I was going to eat next. Why couldn't I just say no to seconds and thirds? When would I start my next diet?

Now I think about food as much as I used to, only the

thoughts have changed. Now, I wonder how full I'll be able to feel tonight. If I risk having just a little bit of sweets will the hot sweats get me? I would like to sit in front of my food and shovel it in like I used to, but now I'm forced to taste it and then pretend it was my whole meal. It's very traumatic to my psyche. My attitude has gone from positive to negative, and the whole world looks kind of black to gray.

Shirley

One day, I saw an ad in a telephone book that advertised "Surgical Control of Weight." I began to seriously consider surgery to control my weight after I called the number and received a videotape of a doctor talking about the three kinds of surgery available at that time.

I signed up, and went to a group meeting where risks were explained and where several women who had the surgery spoke to us about how wonderful their lives were now. They also passed around before and after pictures that were astonishing. Some of the women did not even look like themselves after their faces got thin. My husband had been very skeptical about such a surgery. He accepts me the way I am, which was a reassurance to me that I wanted to do this for myself and not for anyone else. He went to the preoperative meeting with me and, when he saw the difference in the people that were there, he said he'd support me in my decision to go ahead with the surgery.

I had mixed feelings as the weeks passed between my initial call and the surgery. There is a wide gap of time, lasting from three to six months to longer, in which all medical records are gathered, and the insurance companies approve or disapprove of the surgery. It is difficult to wait, especially when you want the surgery done yesterday. I found that every annual event I went to that food was involved in was a cause for mourning. I thought to myself, "This will be the last time you will be able to eat whatever you want at *this* event." I began not watching what I ate so vigilantly as before, because I fully expected that the surgery would take off the weight. Consequently, my clothes became tight as I gained a few pounds. I cannot let myself eat what I want even for one day without gaining weight. However, this only increased my desire to go ahead with the surgery quickly.

Three weeks after I sent in the release of information pages to my former doctors, I called the weight loss center. Five of the sixteen doctors had not yet sent in my records. When I called their offices, two had no record of receiving a permission form, two had quit practicing, and one claimed they just mailed it out that day. I was ready to go ahead, and this delay was disheartening. It meant that it would be at least two more weeks before the center called me to schedule an appointment for a physical and history, and even longer before they would submit a "need" letter to the insurance company and receive approval (or disapproval).

In the meantime, I arranged for the six tests that were listed in the initial packet from the doctor's office which were: abdominal ultrasound, blood chemistry, chest X ray, electrocardiogram, oximetry, and upper GI series. I thought that, if the tests were done prior to my seeing the bariatric doctor, it would speed things up.

There is a lot of conflicting information about weight loss surgery on the Internet. Some say it took up to two years for the insurance to approve the surgery. Others claim that, after surgery, the results were less than a ten-pound loss the first month. You can find positive stories and truly frightening stories on the Internet. I was surprised at the number of people who don't know which procedure they had.

There are also many different programs for postoperative support, from major liquid diets and supplements to one lady who was told to just chew two children's chewable vitamins a day, and that was it. One person claimed that the size of the outlet from the pouch to the lower stomach was a quarter-inch. That's very small. Another woman said hers was a half-inch. That seems more reasonable. I learned later that the calibration instrument is 12 millimeters, which is slightly more than half an inch. I don't know how large the naturally occurring outlet is. The Marlex nylon band around the upper pouch and lower stomach will not allow for expansion of the opening. However, stretching of the upper stomach occurs naturally with larger portions of food, especially if you drink carbonated soda, because of the bubbles.

I finally got all the required documents in to the doctor, and the letter was sent to the insurance company. They received it on Monday and, on Tuesday, we got word that it had been rejected because of a specific exclusion in my insurance policy for gastroplasty. The receptionist from the office called me with the news. Then she said, "I don't know what you want to do now." I had read in their initial papers that their office would support me through the appeals process. I didn't feel very supported. I immediately went to the computer and composed an appeal letter, which I sent on Wednesday. By Friday, I had gotten a letter back from the insurance company saying they denied me the procedure again because of a specific exclusion in the policy. My only hope now is to change insurance at my company's next open enrollment period, or to try to go out of the country. I'm so depressed I could kill myself. I thought there was some hope for me, but now there's none.

Deardra

I am 45 years old. My husband was reluctant when I told him I wanted to have gastric bypass. He wanted me to try to diet again. I told him I was through with diets. All they ever did for me was to add pounds. I weighed 364 before the surgery. I wanted the most radical kind, where they reconnect the intestines and make the stomach smaller. My husband is now very supportive of my decision because he knows how important this is to me. He tells me he loves me the way I am. That's important to me. I wouldn't want to be with someone who didn't love me for myself. I can't wait until I am physically able to do all the activities we dream of.

I have two beautiful children. They don't know quite what to think about this. I'm sure they don't understand, because they love the big "fluffy" mama that I am now. But they are one of my reasons for doing this. I want to be able to go on hikes and bike rides with them, to go to amusement parks and be able to ride the rides. Last time I went to Disney World, I tried a ride, but they made me get off and sit it out. It was totally embarrassing to have to walk back through the crowds after being too big to fasten the belt around me.

I have been overweight all my life. When I was eight years old I went on my first diet. I was just eating salad and meat for dinner. My whole family went on it with me. They all lost weight, and I went from 125 pounds to 98 pounds. But I didn't change my eating habits for good, so I gained the weight back.

First, I want to talk about the prep for surgery. There is medication to help prevent infection. With my surgery, there was also really repugnant stuff to drink to clean out the large intestine. I couldn't stomach this. It was so salty that it made me gag. I was supposed to drink about a gallon of it. I could only manage half of it. They decided to go ahead anyway.

I arrived at the hospital at 5:30 A.M. The nurse took my blood pressure and temperature, and also ordered an enema for me. She started the IV and did the enema.

The anesthesiologist came in and we talked a bit. He ordered something else to take care of the acid in my stomach. He warned me to chug it in one gulp, not to sip. One sip of this stuff and you feel like throwing up.

I walked down to the operating room. They put leggings on me that fill with air, and then deflate, to help keep the circulation going. This helps to prevent blood clots. Then I was out for the count.

I don't remember feeling the esophageal tube until I was back in my room. It was still in. I was in incredible pain, and I pressed the button for more medication. My kids were curled up on the floor with blankets asleep. My mom was on a couch, and my husband on a chair. All of them were asleep. I don't remember them leaving. The second day they took out the catheter and the tube. Now I had to get up and go to the bathroom. I had a bed that basically lifted me to a standing position. It was difficult to walk to the bathroom the first time but after that, it was easier.

Sometime during the second day we found that the medication dispenser hadn't been working. No wonder I was in such pain. The food I was given was like baby food. I did manage some Jell-O and soup. Ice chips were great, and soothed my sore throat. Then I found out that I had a stricture at the junction of the small intestine and stomach. Nothing could get through! I could have starved to death. The doctor did a scope and said there was undigested food just sitting there in my stomach. He tried a procedure that opened the stricture, which kind of worked for a while, but it closed up again, and I had to have another scope. They ended up scoping me about four times, and finally decided I had to go back to surgery to clear it up for good. That was horrible to live through.

The next day the depression hit. I had been off of my Paxil and I didn't feel I could go on. I wished I would've died on the operating table so that I wouldn't have to go through this, the pain was so horrible. Now I have to start over with learning to eat. But, knowing what could happen, I almost don't want to try.

I left for home on the tenth day. Mom drove me. It was a long two-hour drive. The bumps in the road were like mountains. I slept in a recliner for two weeks and I couldn't lie flat because of reflux and pain.

I was having trouble sleeping when I first got home, and I took Benedryl to help me sleep, Darvocet for pain and Pepcid for heartburn. That night I had nightmares. The next day I found out you can't mix those medications.

The first week at home sleep was difficult. I would wake up hourly. Eating was difficult and I threw up a lot. Most mornings I had Cream of Wheat and Popsicles to help with the liquid intake. I tried soups for lunch and dinner. I also tried an egg. Most of what I tried didn't stay down. I was constantly throwing up but, since I had only eaten about a tablespoonful, it was more like spit-up. I carried a towel with me wherever I went because I sometimes couldn't make it to the bathroom.

On Saturday, I went back to the emergency room for IV fluids and blood tests. I was dehydrated and my white blood count was up. So I went back to liquids. I tried to drink in little sips because it would stay down better than if I chugged it.

During the third week at home I started keeping the food down better. I had the dry heaves daily, though. I got the hiccups every time I attempted to eat and, with the stitches, they really hurt. My energy level was low and I got tired easily. The depression was still there, but I tried to fight it. That day's goal was to answer the phone if it rang. I slept off and on until noon. Once out of bed I did answer the phone. The next day a friend was going to drive me around to get out of the house. I wanted to sign up for a class to help me out of the depression.

The sixth week after surgery I found I had lost 37 pounds. That was encouraging, but I didn't quite trust it because, before, I had always gained back the weight. I had a half slice of toast for breakfast, half a burrito for lunch, and frozen yogurt and a Popsicle in the afternoon. For dinner, I had one ounce of chicken, which is about the size of my little finger, and one fish stick, and I didn't throw up. I did actually feel full on that little bit of food. I learned you can't gulp food without chewing it well, like used to, because then the pain hits hard and fast.

I did have a lot of pain, depression, and difficulty eating after my surgery. Other people breeze right though. Not everyone goes through this the same way. I'm looking forward to the day when I feel good again, both mentally and physically. This isn't an effortless change. The food you eat after the surgery is almost like a punishment for a while. When you feel like food is stuck in your throat so much, you get conditioned not to eat, because with eating comes the pain. I was willing to trade my enjoyment of food—and large quantities of it—for a slender body. Not everyone would be satisfied with the trade-off.

After one year I lost 135 pounds, and I'm still losing. I am pleased with the results, although I would like to get below 200 pounds. I have mixed feelings about my body, though. It looks great but I'm really malnourished, and I'm afraid of the future because the long-term statistics haven't really been explored.

Beth

I had the adjustable gastric band procedure on November 12, 1998. It was the best decision I have ever made, and I have not had one minute of regret. I have lost nearly 130 pounds, and am working on the last 20. I believe the reason the surgery worked so well for me was the fact that I was prepared. I researched the surgery, the doctors and the hospital, thoroughly. I also educated myself and my family for the lifestyle changes that would be needed. The more prepared you are, the more successful you will be. I was nervous and anxious about failing on the program, as I have on the hundreds of other plans before this. Remember that this surgery is a tool that you are given. You are in control of it, and need to learn how to use it. Make use of support through the office staff, and through other patients as well.

Wearing size 12–14 clothes, shopping off the racks in regular size departments, fitting into movie theater seats, airplane seats, and rides at amusement parks are just some of the "side effects" of this surgery! Not being sick in over two years, being able to walk three to five miles at a time, and extending my life by being more healthy are some of the other benefits. I was about 250 pounds when I went in, which was about 120 pounds too much for my 5-foot, 2-inch frame. I am now 130 pounds, and have been at this same weight for over five years. I never even think about dieting anymore and am more active than I've ever been.

For me, it was a totally positive experience. But I have a

high tolerance for pain, am very physically active, and I wasn't as huge as some of the people that undergo this procedure. I know of other people who have had a negative experience, and even some who reversed the procedure after a few months of what they termed a "living hell."

Hanna

At the beginning of March, 1997, I weighed around 350 pounds. I had lost some weight prior to this surgery. Usually people gain weight prior to having the surgery. I've been planning this surgery for six months. In November I weighed about 370 pounds. I had just been diagnosed with type II diabetes. I was finding it difficult to walk because of the weight. I also found out in January that I had an umbilical hernia, which could be fixed at the same time as my bypass. I also had stress incontinence that was very annoying. Sometimes I sneezed and wet my pants. At home, this can be managed, but at work it was embarrassing. I was fed up with the waiting period my insurance company imposed and anxious to have it over and done with. I spent the week up until the surgery eating things I thought I might not be able to have afterwards. It was sad to say good-bye to my favorite foods.

I went into the hospital the afternoon before my operation. They did an ECG and a chest X ray that afternoon. A lab technician took a sample of blood. I had a visit from the anesthetist. I was given dinner that evening, and toast and coffee for breakfast in the morning. I didn't get into surgery until 2:30 P.M. because there was someone scheduled before me. The IV was started, and I began to feel very groggy. I couldn't have an epidural for the actual surgery because it would have suppressed my breathing too much, but I did get an epidural in my back for pain relief after the operation. The next thing I knew, it was 7:00 P.M. I was back in my room, and had the IV drip, the epidural and an oxygen mask for the next few days, on and off. At first, I couldn't have anything to eat or drink, but gradually was allowed ice chips and water. I had to be able to drink a reasonable quantity of water before the IV could be removed. Then I was put on a special diet. It was tiny quantities of soft or liquid food. After four days I was well enough to go home.

That was in March of 1997. I didn't have too many complications once I got home. The weight came off really fast during the first three months. By July, I had lost about 80 pounds. I've gone through several sets of clothes. I've started going to the thrift shops and consignment shops for my clothes now. At the consignment shops, I can wear something for a couple of months and then have them resell it for me. I've got quite an account going over there.

It's kind of depressing to see others eating a big meal and to be just as hungry as they are, but only be able to get down half a cup of food. I still get tired easily. That has been my main complaint. I can eat a range of foods, if I make sure to chew well. Most of the time though, I just have soup. It's easier to manage. Even then, I'll occasionally throw it up. I feel rather nauseous if I eat too much and the food gets hung up and won't go through the "hole." I haven't taken any medication for my diabetes since the surgery, and my fasting blood glucose is good. In fact, my random glucose level is 7.5, and that is lower than my fasting level was before the surgery. I saw the doctor and found out my iron levels were low. Since beginning iron replacement therapy some of my energy has come back.

By mid-May of 1998, just 14 months after my surgery, I'd lost 165 pounds and weighed 185—I was still losing, but more slowly than before. I would have considered the surgery successful at 200 pounds, so I feel great about it. The skin on my stomach and legs wasn't very attractive but I could cover that up. I could see my collarbones now, and I liked the shape of my upper torso. People often ask me if I would do it again and the answer is a resounding, "yes."

One thing I would do differently, though, is to have more counseling before, during and after the surgery. There have been times when the changes in my body and my spouse's reaction to them made it very difficult. My husband eventually left me and moved in with someone fatter than I was to begin with. I think he wanted a mother more than a mate and, to him, a big person was more motherly. Someone suggested that the change is almost as dramatic as in a sex-change operation, and it's certainly not far short of that. I needed a counselor to help me work through some of the issues. I was used to turning to food for comfort and that was no longer possible. I wasn't used to facing anger or sadness or fear without shifting those feelings to food.

After two years, my weight settled in at about 160 pounds. Now, I wear a size 12 dress. I'm very happy with how my surgery turned out. However, if I had known then what I know now, I would have been in marriage counseling before, during and after my surgery. Maybe we could have made the marriage work if we had both been willing to work through some difficult issues. Being fat was always the predominant focus of our life together. When I got thinner, my husband couldn't handle the new me, and I wasn't willing to go back to being the way I had been before. But, all in all, I'm happier now than I have ever been. When I see huge people standing at the back of theaters because they are too wide for the seats, or eating salads in restaurants, I'm so sad for them. I want to tell everyone I see about this wonderful thing that happened to me, but I restrain myself. Those kinds of remarks would not have been welcomed by me when I was a fat person, so I have to accept those people in the same way I would have liked to have been accepted myself when *I* was fat.

Ellie

I suffered from high blood pressure and diabetes, joint and back pain, and had very low self-esteem. I rarely left my house and would order everything I needed from nearby markets or the Internet. At the beginning of my story I weighed about 400 pounds. I had tried all the diets; each had led to depression and despair as the weight piled back on. All I thought about was food. If I was on a diet, I was thinking of the food I had left for the day and how much more I really wanted to eat. If I was not on a diet, I was busy stuffing loads of food into my mouth. I could be in control for about two weeks. Then I would go off the wagon and eat like I was making up for lost time. It was like I was addicted to food.

But I wonder how much I would weigh if I had never gone on a diet? My mother was heavy, about 250 pounds, but not obscenely obese as I was. I can't remember that she ever dieted. She seemed to eat a normal amount to me, always less than my dad, but she was still quite heavy for her height, which was 64 inches.

I had my surgery in May of 1998. The surgery itself is kind of a blur. I remember it wasn't pleasant for about three days afterwards, but I went back to work after just a week and a half. I have lost 140 pounds in the last seven months. I feel self-confident and happy for the first time in years. I know I still weigh over 250 pounds, but I feel great. I look in the mirror sometimes and think I see my mother. Since I always admired her, even though she was fat, I can see that people might be able to like me at this weight. I haven't stopped losing weight, and I look forward to actually wearing clothes that are off the rack in a regular-size department.

I have more energy than I've ever had, and can go through the day without taking several mini-naps. I don't even miss the food I used to eat. I think I was always trying to feel full but, although I ate an enormous amount of food, I never felt satisfied. I can remember that sometimes, after eating two normal-size dinners, several desserts, and drinking lots of milk, I would wonder why I didn't feel stuffed. I know that my stomach didn't hold more than eight cups. It seemed to me that it must have missed the button that turns off appetite in normal people. Now, I eat a half a piece of toast and an egg, and I feel full. Well, not exactly full, but I know I can't eat anymore. Not only that, I don't feel hungry again for several hours. It's great!

My knees, back and hips no longer hurt upon exertion. Before surgery, there were times when going to the mailbox at the end of the driveway would tire me out, and I would have to take a nap or a rest before opening the mail. Now, I bound up and down the stairs and can walk for up to an hour without feeling tired. Previously, I had been facing hip replacement surgery in the near future, and possibly knee replacement after that. But those joints no longer seem to be a problem. Taking 140 pounds of pressure off them helped. I have more weight to lose, but I would be content to just get below 200 pounds. That would be half my original body size.

When I hit the 200-pound mark, the doctors removed the sagging "apron" of skin I had around my middle. My weight loss had slowed down considerably by then, and they thought it would be okay to do the "tummy tuck." It was covered by my insurance because it was for "reconstruction," rather than for cosmetic reasons. I feel like a model now. I fit into size 14–16 jeans and haven't done that since the 5th grade. It's made such a difference in my life that I can't imagine why anyone would think twice about doing it.

Suzy

I was approached by a camera team to do a news feature on my surgery for a major network. My story was photographed and published for all the world to see. I'm not sure who exactly funded the surgery, but it didn't cost me anything. Things didn't turn out all hunky-dory like they thought they would. I am 20 years old and have been all the stereotypes: fat, sloppy, introverted, wearing glasses, ugly, bad hair, bad skin—a real piranha as far as life is concerned. No friends, nobody who loved me except, I guess, my mom, in her own way. I weighed about 300 pounds at 5 feet, 8 inches. Since she was kind of fat and lonely, we made a good team. No one bothered us much, and we ate together and watched TV and read romance novels most of the time. She did get on my case sometimes about doing something with my life. I would just roll my eyes and she would drop it. She wasn't really in a position to criticize me, since she was on welfare at the time and had showed me how to get on it once I turned 18.

I had the surgery done in March and, by September, I began to look and feel different than I ever had. I was suddenly looking pretty good. The TV station paid me to get contact lenses, and they had me go to a skin doctor. I suppose they wanted the contrast between the way I had originally looked, and how I was beginning to look, to be dramatic. They even gave me a budget for some new clothes. It was a dream come true. Now there's a TV program called "Extreme Makeovers." I think I was the first, but they didn't call it by that title, and I've noticed that show mainly portrays average-weight people.

Something happened to me on my way to the top of the heap. I started hanging with the wrong crowd. I really had no idea of how to make friends, so I just went along. We did drugs, alcohol, sex, and partied all the time. I felt invincible because I knew I wouldn't get fat no matter what. In a lot of ways I missed my old life. It was kind of gentle and pre-dictable, but my new life was full of adventure, risks, and so-called friends. After the TV show had done it's report on my outcome, I continued to want the clothes, the attention and the money that they had been giving me. But, even at 140 pounds, without any skills or motivation to succeed, I couldn't find a job that paid more than welfare. I turned to prostitu-tion to get money for drugs and alcohol when I wanted them. My pimp was the nicest guy that ever lived when I did what he wanted. When I didn't, he made it real clear what would happen to me if I tried to leave him.

My mom was disgusted with me and told me not to come around anymore. The only friends I had were on the street. So here I am. There are times when I think things aren't so bad, that I'm happy. But I know deep down inside that I would really rather be the old me than the new me. Even though I'm thin and attractive to the world's eyes, in my own eyes I'm uglier than I ever was before all this started. I wish the TV show would come back and do the real story about me and what really happened to my life. It turned out a lot different than any of us thought it would when I agreed to go ahead with weight loss surgery.

Appendix I

Glossary

ADIPOSE: Fat tissue

ADHESION: Scar tissue that unites two body parts or surfaces that are not normally united - for example, when a loop of intestine adheres to the abdominal wall after surgery.

ADIPOSTAT: Located in the hypothalamus it is a mechanism like a thermostat that seeks to maintain weight at a genetically determined level. (also called set-point)

ADJUSTABLE GASTRIC BAND (AGB): A silicone band is placed laparoscopically around the upper portion of the stomach creating a small stomach pouch. This specially designed band has an apparatus on the inside much like an inner tube that can be filled or emptied of water by using a port that is placed just under the skin in the chest or side. Filling the tube with water results in a tighter constriction and slower emptying of the upper stomach pouch into the lower stomach. If too much weight is being lost, the tube can be emptied of some of the water, causing the opening to enlarge and a faster emptying of stomach contents.

AFFERENT LIMB: The unused portion of the small intestine after gastric bypass. The role of the afferent limb is to collect and dispense gastric juices into the newly formed "Y" where the food meets the digestive juices

AFFERENT LIMB SYNDROME: The unused portion of the intestine develops an overgrowth of bacteria. Theoretically tied to autoimmune disorders that may develop after surgery.

ANOREXIANTS (ALSO ANOREXIGENIC): Any food or drug that causes a decrease in appetite.

APPLE-SHAPED: Having extra fat stored around the mid-section of the body and not on the legs and hips. Also associated with visceral fat stores around internal organs.

ATHEROSCLEROSIS: A buildup of fatty deposits (plaque) on the inside of the arteries that narrows the vessels and slows down blood flow. Causes are high blood pressure, smoking, diabetes, elevated cholesterol and triglyceride levels, some drugs and infections. Treatments include: decreasing fat and increasing fiber in the diet, quitting smoking, exercise, daily aspirin dosage and controlling high blood pressure.

AUTOIMMUNE DISORDERS: The patient's immune system attacks other body systems. Some disorders include: rheumatoid arthritis, vitiligo, lupus, ulcerative colitis, and alopecia.

BARIATRIC: The field of medicine concerned with weight loss.

Bariatric surgery: Surgery on the stomach and/or intestines to help people lose weight by altering the normal digestive process.

Bile: A thick, yellow-green fluid that is secreted by the liver and stored in the gallbladder. Bile is released into the intestine to aid in digestion.

Biliopancreatic Diversion (BPD): About 75% of the stomach is removed. Then a gastric bypass surgery is performed. The arm of the small intestines that collects the bile and digestive juices from various organs remains intact. The remaining intestines are reconnected according to a precise formula that takes into account the length of a person's small intestine. It is most often performed with a duodenal switch. See below.

Binge eating: Consuming 3,000 to 15,000+ calories in two hours or less, feeling out of control, and having the problem at least twice a week for six months.

Body Mass Index: A comparison of body weight to height. It correlates strongly to the total percentage of fat in the body. A person with a BMI of 28 or less is generally considered to be of average build. A BMI over 28 is considered overweight. The BMI can be found by multiplying a person's weight by 703 and dividing twice by height in inches. Ex: A person who is 68 inches tall and weighs 150 would figure their BMI like this: 150 X 703 = 105450/68 = 1550.7352/68 = 22.8. This means that approximately 22% of their body is fat tissue, a healthy amount. A BMI of 40 would indicate approximately 40% of the body is fat tissue, an unhealthy amount.

Body Types: A genetic predisposition to having a thin (ectomorph), medium (mesomorph) or heavy (endomorph) body.

Bowel obstruction: Blockage of the intestine by folding, a foreign body, adhesion, narrowing, malformation, inflammation, or tumor. Symptoms are an inability to eliminate feces, pain, and eventually shock.

A. Ileus: Obstruction of the bowel due to it being paralyzed. The bowel is inactive and prohibits the passage of food. It is common following some surgeries. Also called paralytic ileus.

B. Inflammatory bowel disease: A group of chronic intestinal diseases characterized by inflammation of the bowel. Can lead to intestinal stricture which is a narrowing of the passage.

C. Strangulation of the bowel: Obstruction of the bowel due to its twisting back on itself and blocking the passage of food.

Brown fat: Adipose tissue mostly found in infants in whom it forms about 5% of their body weight. It is brown because the cells in it are packed full of cellular organs called mitochondria that are energy factories. It has a rich supply of blood vessels. It is diminished or absent in adulthood.

Bulimia: Binge eating followed by self-induced methods of purging such as vomiting, laxatives, diuretics or excessive exercise.

Comorbidity: The co-existence of two or more disease processes. Common co-morbidities for the obese are: Type II Diabetes, hip and knee arthritis, shortness of breath, insulin resistance, heart disease, high blood pressure, gallstones, sleep apnea, edema of the lower legs, back or disc disease, skin rashes, hiatal hernia.

CONSTIPATION: Inability to eliminate feces, usually due to the lack of water, fiber, or bulk in the stool. Constipation is medically defined as less than three stools per week. Normally when the feces travels to the anus, a large, bulky quantity tends to straighten out the 90-degree angle in which the colon is situated in comparison to the anus. This signals the brain that elimination is necessary. When the bulk is lessened, and the feces is not in a large bulk, but is in small, dry pellets, the physical straightening of the colon does not occur and it is difficult to eliminate the feces from the body. Pellets are caused by lack of water in the stool, which is in turn caused by slow movement through the colon. Other common causes of constipation are: lack of bulk in the diet, disease, medication, laxative abuse, bulimia, bowel obstruction, malformation, lack of motility, surgery, and stress.

COTTAGE CHEESE TEST: A test that gives the functional size of the stomach pouch. A person rapidly eats a small amount of cottage cheese right from the container until they feel full. Then a measured amount of water is poured back into the cottage cheese carton until the level is at its original level. The amount of water poured back into the cottage cheese is the functional size of the stomach pouch.

DIABETES: Type II (90%) diabetes is caused because glucose cannot get into cells. Cells become less responsive to insulin over time (insulin resistance) and in response the pancreas makes more insulin as blood sugar levels rise. When blood sugar levels remain constantly elevated, the pancreas is exhausted and symptoms begin. Type I diabetes (10%) is caused because the pancreas does not make enough insulin so that glucose does not get into cells.

DISTAL BYPASS: A variation of GBP in which approximately 40-60 inches of intestine are left in which calories can be absorbed. The most radical of the bypass surgeries, it carries the greatest risk for malnutrition.

DUMPING SYNDROME: A group of symptoms that occur when a person has a high sugar load following gastric bypass. These sugars are usually absorbed in the duodenum which is now bypassed. The sugars enter the jejunum or the ileum that are not used to absorbing simple sugars. When the body senses the sugar level rising, it dumps insulin to handle the load. This dramatically lowers available blood sugar. Symptoms include cramps, nausea, palpitations, diarrhea, dizziness and a sense of impending doom.

DUODENAL ULCER: A hole in the lining of the duodenum, which is the first part of the small intestine. Due to gastric acid wearing through the lining of the duodenum, often related to the H. pyloridis bacteria.

DUODENUM: The first part of the small intestine consisting of the pyloric valve, which is the connection point to the stomach, and extending about twelve inches to the jejunum. In Greek, duo + den means 2 + 10. The duodenum is approximately 12 finger widths or inches long.

DUODENAL SWITCH (DS): The duodenal switch is the same as the biliopancreatic diversion with the major difference being that approximately 1-2 inches of the duodenum is left in place below the pylorus sphincter.

DUODENAL ULCER: A hole in the lining of the duodenum (which is the first portion of the small intestine) caused by erosion of the lining by acidic juices. Associated with the H. pyloridis bacteria.

EATING DISORDER: Bulimia, anorexia, binging or food obsessions that cause a person to be thinking about food most of the time.

ESOPHAGUS: The tube-like structure that carries food from the mouth to the stomach. At the bottom of the esophagus, a ring of muscle relaxes to let food into the stomach. When this sphincter does not function normally, and remains open, juices full of acid from the stomach splash back up into the esophagus producing heartburn.

FECAL INCONTINENCE: The inability of the anal nerves and muscles to control the emptying of the bowel.

FOBI POUCH OPERATION (FPO): Originally created by Dr. Matthias Fobi for people who did not lose enough weight with a banded procedure but already had the Marlex mesh band or Silastic ring around the upper part of the stomach. The operation was converted to a bypass and the band was left in place. It also refers to an initial bypass operation in which a band or ring is put in place, limiting the rate that the small pouch can empty.

GALLSTONES: Too much cholesterol in the gallbladder. Caused by the liver excreting too much cholesterol or the bile being out of balance and not dissolving the cholesterol that is excreted. The sticky particles of cholesterol adhere to one another eventually forming larger gallstones.

GASTRIC BALLOON: A small balloon is placed in the stomach through the mouth and esophagus. It is inflated after placement. The balloon takes up room in the stomach and restricts the amount that can be eaten.

GASTRIC BYPASS (GBP): A surgical procedure which involves cutting the stomach in two to create a small stomach pouch and then bypassing the rest of the stomach and half to three quarters of the small intestine. This reduces the amount of fat and calories the body can absorb.

GASTRIC REFLUX: The stomach contents combined with stomach acid regurgitate back up into the esophagus causing inflammation and damage to the esophagus, larynx and lungs. Also called GERD Gastroesophageal reflux disease.

GASTROINTESTINAL: Pertaining to all or some of the organs of the digestive tract, from the mouth to the anus.

GASTROPLASTY: Stomach surgery.

HALITOSIS: Bad breath.

HERBAL REMEDIES: Substances found in nature and deemed a food substance, therefore not under the control of the FDA.

HERNIA: Protrusion of tissue through the wall of the cavity where it is usually contained. A common occurrence after weight loss surgery is a hernia where the newly configured bowels are joined.

HIATAL HERNIA: Part of the upper stomach protrudes through the diaphragm causing heartburn and esophagitis.

HIGH BLOOD PRESSURE: Also called hypertension, it is a condition in which the pressure of the blood in the arteries is too high. No specific cause is found in 95% of cases. It is treated with exercise, limiting salt, losing weight, and medication.

HOMEOSTASIS: The tendency of the body to remain the same. In a state of equilibrium, the body remains relatively constant and resists weight loss efforts by increasing hunger when food is restricted.

HOSPITAL ACQUIRED INFECTION: An infection caught while hospitalized. Various antibiotics used in hospitals are different from outside and certain bacteria become resistant to them, increasing the risk of infection from them while in the hospital. Also called nosocomial infections, they are serious and difficult to treat.

HYPERPARATHYROIDISM: Too much calcium in the blood. This can cause bone to dissolve and leave calcium deposits in the kidneys.

HYPERGLYCEMIA: A condition in which there is too much sugar in the blood.

HYPOXIA: Inadequate supply of oxygen in arterial blood and insufficient delivery to cells and organs so that normal function cannot be maintained.

ILEUM: The last part of the small intestine extending from the jejunum to the large bowel.

IMPLANTABLE GASTRIC STIMULATION SYSTEM (IGS): A pacemaker for the stomach. A small implantable battery pack is implanted under the skin and a wire extends to the vagus nerve of the stomach. It provides electrical stimulation to the nerve which is said to lessen hunger signals. It is undergoing clinical trials in the United States in 2004 but is widely available in Europe. Manufactured by Transneuronix.

INSULIN RESISTANCE: The diminished ability of cells to respond to the action of insulin in transporting glucose from the bloodstream into muscle cells. It is as if insulin is "knocking" on the door of the muscle. Normally the muscle hears the knock and lets the glucose in. With insulin resistance, the muscle cannot hear the knocking of the insulin and cannot utilize the glucose for energy. The pancreas makes more insulin and causes a louder "knock." Eventually the pancreas produces far more insulin than normal, the muscles are still resistant, and blood glucose levels are constantly in the hyperglycemic range.

INSURANCE POLICY EXCLUSION: A denial of insurance coverage due to a specific exclusion. Sometimes listed for weight loss efforts and surgery. This is the most difficult insurance denial to fight unless it can be proven that the insurance company buried or failed to list this exclusion in its policy.

IRON DEFICIENT ANEMIA: Lack of iron in the blood. Iron is necessary to make hemoglobin, the key molecule in red blood cells responsible for the transport of oxygen. In iron deficient anemia, the red blood cells are small and pale. Recommended amounts of iron are 15 mg per day for women and 10 mg per day for men.

INTERNATIONAL SIZE ACCEPTANCE ASSOCIATION: A society dedicated to eliminating sizism, dieting, weight loss surgery and any other practice that places obese persons in a different category than the norm. They believe that persons of all weights should be accepted for who they are.

JEJUNUM: The second part of the small intestine extending from the duodenum to the ileus.

JEJUNO-ILEAL BYPASS (JIB): The original "stomach stapling" performed in the 70's and 80's in which the person's stomach was stapled so that a smaller amount of food could be eaten. It also encompassed bypassing all of the small intestine except for one or two feet. There was a high mortality rate and a high percentage of patients suffered from severe side effects such as malnutrition and diarrhea. Patients often developed fatal liver disease.

LAPAROSCOPY: Surgery done without an open incision. Small incisions are made that allow surgical instruments and a slender illuminated optical or fiber optic camera into the body cavity. Surgery is done by remote control.

LEAN MUSCLE MASS: That portion of the body consisting of muscle, organs, skeletal system, blood vessels, lymphatic system, etc. minus body fat. Most accurately determined by hydrostatic (underwater) weighing.

LIPECTOMY: The process of surgically removing fat tissue from the body by cutting it off.

LIPOSUCTION: The process of removing fat tissue from problem areas on the body using a vacuum system and small incisions of 1/4 to 1 inch.

LIVER: A large internal organ that processes nearly every nutrient we need to make the nutrients usable by other body parts. Enzymes and bile salts made in the liver are sent through a tube and stored in the gallbladder and sent via another tube (the bile duct) to be emptied into the duodenum.

LOOP GASTRIC BYPASS: Same as the mini gastric bypass.

LUPUS: A disease of the skin that can spread to other organs. An inflammatory condition caused by an autoimmune reaction. The body's tissues are attacked by its own immune system. Can cause rash, photosensitivity, ulceration of mucus membranes and swollen, tender joints.

LUX: Lux is the international unit of illumination. A home with the lights on at night usually has from 50–150 lux. A brightly lit office has 200–400 lux. A bright day has 50,000 to 80,000 lux and a cloudy day around 7,000 lux. Bright light affects melatonin, a hormone that regulates sleep and serotonin.

MALABSORPTION: The body is unable to absorb all the calories it ingests due to artificial constraints such as re-configuring the bowel.

MALNUTRITION: A condition caused by a failure to eat or to absorb the foods needed to maintain proper health. Most gastric bypass patients suffer from some form of malnutrition and need constant monitoring.

MARLEX MESH BAND: A reinforced band that inhibits stretching of the small opening between the small stomach pouch and the larger stomach.

MEDIAL GASTRIC BYPASS: The middle portion of the small intestines is used as the connection point for the arms of the small intestine to join together. Of an approximate total length of 20 feet, the junction leaves about 6–10 feet in which to absorb calories.

METABOLISM: The whole range of biological processes that occur within the body that break down food molecules and transform them into energy. Also refers to the body's ability to build the substances it needs from the food we eat.

MINI-GASTRIC BYPASS: The intestine is not severed and reconnected as in the gastric bypass, but after leaving the small upper pouch, it is looped back and reconnected to the small upper pouch so that acids and bile have a chance to get into the pouch and even the esophagus, often creating havoc with stomach and esophageal linings.

MORBID-OBESITY: One hundred pounds or more over the recommended weight on the Metropolitan height-weight chart. Having a BMI of 40–50.

MUSCLE ATROPHY: Wasting away of muscle and a decrease in muscle mass. Atrophy begins in as little as 24 hours when a person is not moving about, such as after surgery.

NEUROTRANSMITTER: A messenger of neurological information from one cell to another by a chemical process. Common neurotransmitters are norepinephrine, serotonin, and dopamine.

OBESITY: Having a BMI of over 30 is the precise measure of obesity subscribed to by the NIH. Obesity is caused by a variety of factors, including: sedentary lifestyle, over-eating, over production of hunger hormones, genetics, high-fat/low fiber diets, a diet high in processed and fast foods, and yo-yo dieting.

OFF-LABEL USE: Prescribing medications for other than their intended use. Sometimes patients and physicians will notice that medications developed for a particular disorder actually help with other disorders as well.

OSTEOMALACIA: Softening of bone because of the depletion of calcium and vitamin D. Commonly called rickets.

OSTEOPOROSIS: Thinning of the bone mass because of the depletion of calcium and bone protein. New bone is not created as fast as old bone is broken down.

PANCREAS: Makes digestive chemicals that break down food and hormones such as insulin that allow cells to use glucose.

PEAR-SHAPED: Having extra fat stored on the hips and thighs.

PROTEIN REQUIREMENTS: The Recommended Dietary Allowance is 44 grams a day for the average woman and 56 grams for the average man. However, this is for individuals whose digestive system is not traumatized by surgery. Recommended protein intake for post WLS patients is between 60-80 grams per day and requires supplemental protein drinks.

PROXIMAL GASTRIC BYPASS: The bypass procedure that reconnects the intestine closest to the original stomach. The junction of the two arms of the small intestines are joined above the middle of the remaining small intestine leaving the longest arm for food absorption, usually greater than 10 feet and sometimes as much as 15 feet. There is a lessened chance of malnutrition with the proximal bypass. Weight loss is also less than with the medial or distal bypass.

PULMONARY EMBOLISM: The obstruction of the pulmonary artery or a branch of it leading to the lungs by a blood clot, usually from the leg, causing sudden closure of the vessel. 10-15% of patients with pulmonary embolism die.

RESTRICTIVE SURGERY: Surgery designed to limit the amount of food one can eat at a time to 3–9 ounces on average.

ROUX-EN-Y GASTRIC BYPASS: The same as the gastric bypass in which the stomach is cut in two and then the rest of the stomach and one half to three quarters of the small intestine is bypassed so that calories are not absorbed. The Y is the shape of the artificial joining of the intestines. One arm of the Y carries the food portion and one arm carries the gastric juices and bile. They join together at an artificial juncture and then move into the large bowel.

SEPSIS: Commonly called a "blood stream infection." The presence of bacteria or other organisms in the blood or other tissue. Causes fever, chills, malaise, low blood pressure and cloudy thinking.

SEROMA: Bacteria gets into a wound, usually from surgery and develops an infection. It may need to be drained more than once.

SILASTIC RING: A small ring that inhibits stretching of the opening between the small stomach pouch and the larger stomach.

SIZE-ISM: Discrimination based on a person's size. Fat people are thought to be lazy, unmotivated, clumsy, less intelligent, unsanitary, and gluttonous.

SLEEP APNEA: Obstructive sleep apnea occurs because the throat collapses during sleep causing the individual to stop breathing for a short time and then snort and gasp for breath. People wake up briefly each time breathing stops and then fall asleep again, never knowing they have awakened. It is common among the obese

SOMATOFORM PERSONALITY: A tendency to manifest physical complaints because of psychological stress. Examples would be getting a debilitating stomachache before giving an oral report or waking up with a headache because a difficult day at work awaits and then calling in sick.

STOMACH: The place where food goes after leaving the esophagus. It begins the process of digestion by softening proteins and breaking down food molecules with hydrochloric acid and pepsin. It usually holds from 4–6 cups of food but can be distended to hold 8–12 cups in a chronic overeater. There is some evidence that the size of the stomach somewhat dictates the hunger level of the person. People with larger stomachs create more hunger hormones than people with smaller stomachs.

STOMACH POUCH: After resecting the stomach it is the small remaining receptacle where food goes from the esophagus. Usually holds 3 to 9 ounces of food.

STOMACH ULCER: A hole in the lining of the stomach that has been eroded by acidic juices. Often related to the *H. pyloridis* bacteria in the stomach.

SUBCUTANEOUS: Just under the skin, as in subcutaneous fat.

SUGAR SUBSTITUTES: Saccharin, aspartame, acesulfame, and sucralose are the major sugar substitutes in the U.S. They have a sweet flavor but no calories.

SUPER-ABSORBER: Having a combination of genes that makes it likely the body will hold onto fat stores. Such a person will experience renegade weight gain at several times in their life. It is difficult to lose weight as a super-absorber.

SUPER-MORBIDLY OBESE: Two-hundred or more pounds overweight and having a BMI of 50 or more. A BMI of 50 would mean that approximately 50% of the body mass is fat tissue.

THERMOGENIC: Any food, drug or activity that boosts metabolism. With thermogenic substances there is an increase in perspiration, blood flow, heart rate and movement of food through the digestive system.

TITRATION: Increasing the dose of a medication over time.

THYROTOXICOSIS: An excessive amount of thyroid hormone circulating in the blood because of an overactive thyroid or inflammation of the thyroid gland. Symptoms include increased heart rate, irregular heartbeat, weight loss, depression and fuzzy thinking.

VERTICAL BANDED GASTROPLASTY: Creation of a small stomach receptacle within the larger stomach. A line of staples is placed vertically along the stomach wall and a band restricting the volume of food leaving the small stomach is placed at the bottom. This allows the contents of the smaller stomach to drain slowly into the remaining stomach.

WEIGHT LOSS SURGERY (WLS): Surgery to control weight either with restrictive changes in the configuration of the stomach or malabsorption techniques by modifying the intestinal tract.

YO-YO DIETING: Losing and regaining weight multiple times usually resulting in higher and higher ending weights.

Appendix II

Sample Weight-Loss Surgery Release Form

The following sample weight loss surgery release form is given to patients. Similar release forms are used by several doctors, surgeons, and insurance companies across the United States. Each patient is asked to read it carefully and sign each section before surgery.

Obesity Surgery: Considerations

Obesity is clearly an alarming health problem in the United States. Not only is the total number of obese individuals increasing, but also the age of onset of obesity is decreasing. Younger and younger individuals have become morbidly obese, and are even experiencing adult-type diabetes and heart disease at an unusually early age. Clearly the health habits of Americans are deadly. Individuals who are obese typically feel that they are going to die any minute simply because of how much they weigh. They may feel they are discriminated against because of their weight. There is occasionally an underlying feeling that something drastic or violent needs to be done to their body, in order to tame the fact that it is out of control. In their frustration, these individuals place their physician in the position of the bad guy if he doesn't find them a good surgeon for the procedure. However, they must realize that the decision to use surgery to lose weight is not a patient decision. It is a medical decision. You may know people who have had surgery for their weight, and everything has gone fine afterwards. They tell you that it was the best decision they ever made. They urge you to get the same procedure. However, it is also not their decision to make. It is a medical decision, taking you and your current mental and physical health into account. Obesity surgery is not strictly preventive. It is a medical treatment. It is a choice between two options, neither of which is ideal. Patients often believe that the surgery is a preventive therapy. This is untrue; preventive therapy would have kept them from becoming obese in the first place. Obesity is a sickness, and surgery is only one treatment for it. It may not even be the best one, or have the best outcome.

Read and Understood

Surgeons will tell their patients that their problem is a genetic one, and that their only choice is to have this surgery. While genetics play a role, this reasoning is flawed. It happens to be true that all races within the United States have an increased risk of obesity over their genetic counterparts within other countries.

Europeans are more likely to be obese in the United States than Europe. Asians are more likely to be obese in the United

States than their country of origin. Likewise, African-Americans, Hispanics, Pacific Islanders, and East Indians, all are likely to be heavier in this country. America is a bad place to live if you do not wish to be obese. Obesity involves complex physiology. Do not blame the lack of a cure on your doctor. Instead, blame a food industry that wants your money and will "feed" you anything to get it. We have seen patients go to other countries to live for a while and lose weight while there. We have seen patients come from these other countries and immediately begin to put on weight.

Read and Understood

_____

If you believe that having this surgery will mean that you do not have to change what you eat, you are mistaken. If it works correctly, this surgery changes WHAT you eat, not just how much. All patients eat less. Typically, those individuals who find that they can eat anything they want after they have the surgery, are the same individuals who either lose little weight or who eventually gain the weight back.

Read and Understood

_____

If you believe this surgery will restore you to complete and normal health, you are mistaken. You are trading one nutrition problem for another. Obesity alone does not necessarily kill you. You need to understand that, when researchers do studies on the obese and find that they are more likely to die, this does not necessarily mean that how much they weigh is what killed them. Obesity is a symptom; it is just as likely that _what_ the obese ate killed them, and also happened to make them heavy at the same time. Doctors who tell you "Just eat less" oversimplify the problem. You don't need to eat less, you need to eat *differently*. This is the real reason obesity surgery works for some people. The changes they should have made without surgery are forced on them by side effects of the surgery. You will actually do best if fat and sugar make you sick after the procedure. Do not think you know better because you had a friend who had the surgery, who did well despite eating whatever they wanted. They are the exception. Given enough time, they will probably put most of the weight back on.

Read and Understood

_____

Keep In Mind: Slender individuals can have adult diabetes. Slender individuals can have heart attacks. Slender individuals can develop arthritis and have joint problems. Slender individuals can have strokes and develop cancer. If obese individuals have these problems more commonly than the slender, it is because the same bad health habits don't happen to cause obesity in some of those individuals "fortunate" enough to be slender no matter what they eat. They may be slender, but they could very likely die just as early in life as someone who is overweight.

Read and Understood

_____

As doctors, we are nearly always told, "I am willing to take the risk of dying from this surgery because it is better than going on like this" and "I don't want to be a model. I just want my health back".

All but a very few of these people later cry about the fact that they did not lose all the weight they wanted to lose. They are unhappy even though their health is improved. Many of them come back and want other cosmetic tune-ups like liposuction, tummy tucks and skin removal from their arms. Several insurance companies do not have a cosmetic surgery benefit. Save some of the money you are not spending on food for these elective procedures.

Read and Understood

_____

Gastric surgery for weight loss causes nutritional deficiency in nearly 100 percent of the individuals who have it done. The most common deficiencies are Vitamin B12, Iron, Calcium, Magnesium, Carotene (beta-carotene and other carotene vitamins) and potassium. In the beginning, patients will faithfully get their vitamin B12 shots and take their vitamins. After a while, they flatter themselves that they are healthy and just like anyone else. They discontinue getting checkups. This is risky. A recent follow-up study done on gastric bypass patients showed that, even 10 years later, there were severe nutritional deficiencies. You will NEVER be normal after weight loss surgery. NEVER.

Read and Understood

_____

If you have mental health issues like depression, anorexia, or bulimia, you must not hide these problems. If you have any mental health history of any kind, you must report it to the doctor who may refer you for this surgery. Initialing here signifies that you have reported any of these problems. The insurance company cannot be responsible for what you have not disclosed.

Read and Understood

_____

If you have hidden or unreported problems with alcohol or drug abuse, you must report these prior to the surgery. The surgery could very likely kill you if this is true.

Read and Understood

_____

If you have pre-existing nutritional deficiencies, or vitamin deficiencies because of poor eating habits, you must report these, and they must be corrected before surgery is even considered. It is not always possible to correct deficiencies once the surgery is performed. An example would be iron deficiency anemia.

Read and Understood

_____

If you are a candidate for surgery, you must take either a high-quality liquid vitamin or chewable vitamin, with a complete listing of vitamins and minerals, for the rest of your life. Flintstones chewable vitamins are one example. There are three or more versions of these vitamins, and you need to carefully check for the one with the longer list of nutrients. Unless your vomiting is severe, take these daily, even if you occasionally regurgitate or vomit food. If you are regurgitating and/or vomiting, but are able to swallow any water or sip anything at all, you should be able to safely chew and swallow a small vitamin. Often patients complain that they do not like the flavor of these vitamins. Sorry, you must take them anyway.

Read and Understood

A complete inability to eat, or an ongoing problem with vomiting, is a dangerous situation. Fasting for more than three to four days is dangerous. Do not let a problem like this go on more than a day before seeking medical attention. Carefully document what you are able to eat and report it to the health care provider who sees you. Up to 30 percent of individuals develop ulcers where their intestines will join their stomach. This can cause vomiting and abdominal pain. Other more serious internal problems, like bowel strangulation, perforation, infection of the inner abdomen, and gallstones can cause the same thing. Seek medical help, and make it clear to the provider that you have had gastric surgery. If possible, it is best to go back to the surgeon, if the surgery was recently performed. Remember, this is the surgery YOU asked for. If you wait days or weeks to seek medical help, we cannot be responsible for the complications or nutritional problems that occur.

Read and Understood

You should be aware that, as nutritional science advances, we are discovering that there is more to food and health than vitamins, minerals, fiber, protein, carbohydrates and fat. Deficiencies in these nutrients result in rapid health effects that make diagnosis easy. Nutrition science is now moving into new areas involving other more obscure chemicals in plants that have more subtle and long-term effects on health. The subtlety of their effects makes them harder to find, and their benefits more difficult to document. Most health studies are not done long enough to discover all outcomes. As these new substances are located and understood, it will probably emerge that our stomachs have to be a given size just to take them all in. Because of this surgery, you will not be able to do so. Biologically, we have the GI tract we have for a reason. Changing its size and conformation is purely experimental.

Read and Understood

Fruits, grains, vegetables, beans, nuts and wild animals (that were tough and hard to catch), existed on this planet long before farm machinery, stockyards, commercial animal-processing plants, and refineries. While what you do is your business, as far as your body is concerned, you do not have the right to eat abnormally. Your body chemistry will not adapt to junk food just because you wish it to, and this surgery does not make junk food good for you either. Abuse your body and you lose. Chips, sugar, sodas, cookies, cakes, pudding, fast food, snacks, fried foods and excessive fat intake did not exist for human consumption before the last 75–100 years. What we consider food in this country is so different from what humans used to eat, we are almost certain to get sick on it as well as to gain weight. Gastric bypass does NOT enable you to eat these foods and be healthy anyway. Normal weight is NOT all that is necessary to be healthy. When your stomach is the size of a teacup, and your small intestine arranged to cause malabsorption, you cannot eat poor quality food. You need every opportunity you have to even *begin* to get the nutrition you need. Gastric bypass creates malabsorption.

You will not absorb all you eat because of what has been done to you. Gastric bypass makes poor eating habits no longer an option. We can't come check your cupboards. This is your responsibility.

Read and Understood

_____

Complications include, but are not limited to, infection, rupture, strangulation of the bowel, ulcers, non-healing of the wound, hernia at the incision, excessive skin, abdominal pain, vomiting, nutritional deficiencies, depression, arthritis, gas, diarrhea, hair loss, gallstones, bone demineralization, menstrual changes, headaches, weight regain, body odor, bad breath, reflux, heartburn, pulmonary embolisms, heart attack or stroke, or blood clots, as well as death from the surgery itself. Remember that those who had the surgery, and say it was the best thing that ever happened to them, are the ones who are alive to tell you their side of the story. You're getting only part of the picture, no matter what you learned from a friend, a TV news magazine, or on the Internet.

Read and Understood

_____

I have been given a copy of this.

Date_____

Signed_____

Witness_____

Appendix III

Helpful Web Sites

www.aboutsurgicalweightloss.com
www.advancedobesitysurgery.com
www.amedeo.com
www.asbs.org
www.belighter.com
www.beyondchange-obesity.com
www.clos.net
www.compasswls.com
www.duodenalswitch.com
www.fhshealth.org
www.foodanddiet.com
www.hotelveramar.com/
    obesity_surgery
www.laparoscopy.net
www.lapband.co.uk
www.lapband.com
www.lbsremoved.com
www.mygastricbypass.com
www.obesityhelp.com
www.obesehelp.net
www.obesitylawyer.com
www.obesitymd.org
www.obesity-online.com

www.obesitysurger-info.com
www.obesitysurgery.com
www.pubmedcentral.nih.gov
www.pulseamerica.org
www.realage.com
www.spotlighthealth.com
www.surgicalteam.com
www.vh.org/adult/patient/
    surgery/weightcontrolsurgery
www. weightlosssurgerycoach.com
www.wlsfriends.com

Appendix IV

Weight Loss Surgery Quiz

Weight loss surgery is a life-changing decision. It should be considered only as a last resort, when health is threatened and the only alternative is a miserable existence. However, some of the ramifications of the surgery are themselves miserable to deal with for the rest of your life.

This quiz is designed to help you determine whether or not weight loss surgery would be a good option for you. Seriously consider your response to each question on a "good" day, as well as on a day when you are feeling low. Then pursue weight loss surgery only if you truly feel you would be better off with the very real consequences of the surgery as explained in other sections of this book.

Key: **A** = False **B** = Occasionally **C** = Frequently **D** = True

1. I cannot do the things I used to do because of my weight.
   A   B   C   D
2. I would be more active if I were thin.
   A   B   C   D

3. I have significant health problems because of my weight.

   A   B   C   D

4. I have seriously tried dieting for more than one month at least five times.

   A   B   C   D

5. I have lost more than 50 pounds and gained it back.

   A   B   C   D

6. My parents or grandparents died prematurely partly because of their weight.

   A   B   C   D

7. I have successfully handled life-altering changes in my life without getting depressed.

   A   B   C   D

8. My life would be happier if I were thin.

   A   B   C   D

9. My life would be worth living if I were thin.

   A   B   C   D

10. I feel that my immediate family would be better off without me as I am today.

    A   B   C   D

11a. (If married) If I were thin, my partner would love me more than they do now.

    N/A   A   B   C   D

11b. (If unmarried) If I were thin, I would have an easy time finding someone to care for me.

    N/A   A   B   C   D

12. If I were thin, I would alter my lifestyle so drastically that others would not be able to recognize me.

    A   B   C   D

14. I can name three things I <u>cannot</u> do because of my weight.

    1. _____

2. _____

3. _____

A   B   C   D

15. If there were no mirrors in society, and no one cared how I looked, I could be happy with the way I am right now.

A   B   C   D

16. There are activities I avoid because of my appearance.

A   B   C   D

17. I have some eating problems that I don't think most people have, such as bulimia and/or bingeing more than 3,000 calories at one time several times a month.

A   B   C   D

18. I have been told, or wondered if I have, an obsessive-compulsive personality.

A   B   C   D

19. I have some obsessive-compulsive indicators such as:

alcohol abuse

child abuse

drugs

excessive cleaning

flashes of rage

hoarding of food or junk

pornography

promiscuity

shopaholism

shoplifting

workaholism

A   B   C   D

20. I have been overweight since childhood.

A   B   C   D

21. *For women only:* I was unable to lose my pregnancy weight within the first year after childbirth.

A   B   C   D

22. *For men only:* I seemed to gain most of my weight before the age of 30.

A   B   C   D

23. *For teens only:* I don't believe I eat too much compared to other teens I know.

A   B   C   D

Scoring   score_____

Questions 1 through 8	A = 0 B = 5 C = 10 D = 15
Questions 9 through 18	A = 15 B = 10 C = 5 D = 0
Questions 19 through 22	A = 0 B = 5 C = 10 D = 15

Over 250 points: This surgery may be the only way to control your weight, but its life-altering ramifications should be considered carefully. Weight loss surgery will affect your eating style, and drastically limit your food choices for the rest of your life.

200–250 points: The risks and problems associated with this surgery may outweigh the benefits at this point in your life. Positive lifestyle changes, such as learning a new skill, starting a competitive sport such as tennis, golf or volleyball, or starting a "Gratitude Journal" (featured on the television program OPRAH) will be beneficial to you. Consider this surgery only when health-related issues are making your life miserable.

150–200 points: You are generally healthy, and have a good attitude about yourself and about life in general. It is worth trying another serious exercise program, and making some small changes in regard to your diet before choosing to undergo any of these drastic surgeries. Health issues should be the only reason for opting to have one of these procedures.

100–150 points: This surgery is not magic, it won't make you more active, change your lifestyle or make you happy if you are not already happy with yourself as you are. There may be some psychological issues that you need to explore before committing to this surgery.

Under 100 points: This surgery is not for you at this time.

Note

If you answered *true* for number 15, you should consider that your feelings about yourself are more society induced, and do not actually have to have an impact on how you feel about yourself. In other words, you are having a negative impact on yourself when you don't need to.

If you answered true to numbers 17, 18, or 19, you should know that having this surgery will exacerbate your impulse-control problems. Food has been a coping mechanism that has sometimes worked in the past. Without food to turn to, your compulsive traits may surface in a way that is more harmful than overeating was. If you seriously consider this surgery, have the wisdom to participate in ongoing psychological counseling at the same time.

Appendix V

Success Stories

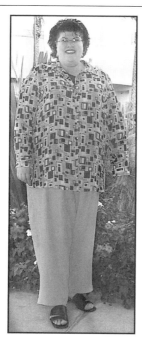 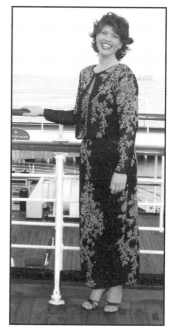

Name: Tammara
Beginning weight: 314
End weight: 149

Pounds lost: 165
Height: 5'6"
Type of surgery: GBP

On the following three pages are five success stories that the author collected while researching this book. For each person, we've included a "before" and an "after" photograph as well as information about how much weight each one lost and what specific type of surgery he or she underwent.

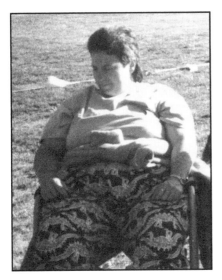 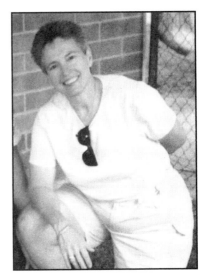

Name: Celia
Beginning weight: 274
End weight: 170

Pounds lost: 105
Type of surgery: RNYGBP

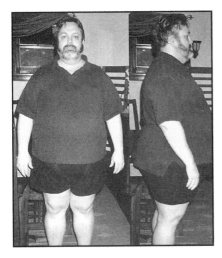 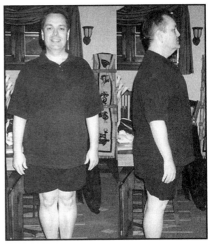

Name: Kenton
Beginning weight: 348
End weight: 220

Pounds lost: 128
Height: 5'7"
Type of surgery: RNYGBP

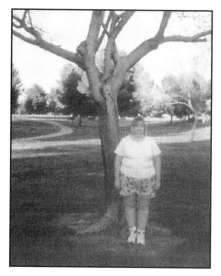

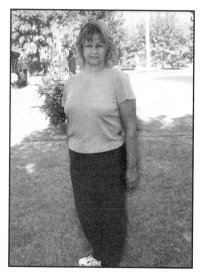

Name: Katie
Beginning weight: 264
End weight: 169

Pounds lost: 95+
Height: 5'4"
Type of surgery: Laproscopic
GBP

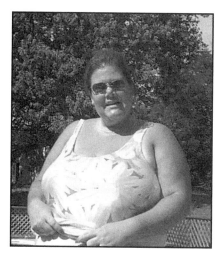

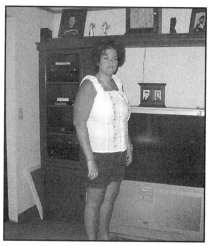

Name: Mischelle
Beginning weight: 320
End weight: 175

Pounds lost: 145
Height: 5'8"
Type of surgery: GBP

End Notes

CHAPTER 1

1. "Rationale for the Surgical Treatment of Morbid Obesity." *American Society for Bariatric Surgery*. Updated Nov. 29, 2001. www.asbs.org/html/rationale.

2. Ibid.

3. Mason, Edward E. M.D. Ph.D. "Vertical Gastroplasty." *IBSR Newsletter Spring 2002*: Vol. 17 No. 1. www.surgery.uiowa.edu/ibsr.

4. Munk, Valen B. "Long-term effects of gastric banding for weight reduction." Haugesund, Norway. *Tidsskr Nor Laegeforen.* 2000 June 30; 120(17): 1995-6.

5. Fox, Ross M.D. "Vertical Gastric Band," "Adjustable Gastric Band," and "Gastric Bypass Surgery." www.drrossfox.com/ vertbnd.html/ adjsbnd.html/gastrby.html, 2000.

6. Ibid.

7. Melinek J, E Livingston, G Cortina, MC Fishbein. "Autopsy Findings Following Gastric Bypass Surgery for Morbid Obesity." *Arch Pathol Lab Med.* 2002 Sept; 126(9): 1091–5.

8. Hell E, KA Miller, MK Moorehead et al. "Evaluation of health status and quality of life after bariatric surgery: Comparison of standard Roux-en-Y gastric bypass, vertical banded gastroplasty and laparo-

scopic adjustable silicone gastric banding." *Obes Surg 2000;* 10:214–19.

9. Sannen I, J Himpens, G Leman. "Causes of dissatisfaction in some patients after AGB," Dept. of Surgery, Dendermonde, Belgium. *Obes Surg 2001.* Oct; 11(5): 605-8.

10. Clark, Wesley Jr. M.D.. *RNY vs DS.* 2003. obesitysurgery-info.com/rnyvsds-wesclark.htm.

11. Strickland, Shelly. *Gastric Electrical Stimulation by the Gastric Pacemaker.* 2003. www.bae.ncsu.edu/research/blanchard/ gastricpacer.

12. Bioenterics Intragastric Balloon (BIB). 2003. www.aprime.com/En/ CA_Balloons.htm.

13. Mason, Edward. E. M.D. Ph.D. "Mortality in Obesity Surgery." *Spring 2003 IBSR Newsletter* Vol. 18 No. 1. www.surgery.uiowa.edu/ibsr.

14. Clark, Wesley Jr. M.D. *Regarding Surgical Mortality Statistics.* 2003. obesi-tysurgery-info.com/surgicalmortalitygwclark.htm.

15. Flanagan, Latham M.D., *The Cottage Cheese Test.* June 2000. www.sabariatric.com/cottage_cheese_test.htm.

CHAPTER 2

1. Mason, Edward E. M.D. Ph.D. "Mortality in Obesity Surgery." *Spring 2003 IBSR Newsletter* Vol. 18 No. 1. www.surgery.uiowa.edu/ibsr.

2. Woodward, Bryan G. *The Complete Guide to Obesity Surgery.* Victoria, B.C.: Trafford Publishers, 2001.

3. Posjasek, Jill. *Ten Habits of Naturally Slim People.* Chicago: Contemporary Books, 1997.

4. *Build Study 1979.* Chicago: Society of Actuaries and Association of Life Insurance Medical Directors of America, 1980.

5. Gaesser, Glenn. A. Ph.D. *Big Fat Lies, The Truth About Your Weight and Your Health.* New York: Fawcett-Columbine Books, 1996.

6. Ibid.

7. Ernsberger, Paul Ph.D. "Surgery for Weight Loss: Comparison of Risk and Benefit." *Obesity and Health* (renamed *Healthy Weight Journal*). March 1991.

8. Fitzgerald, Faith, M.D. "The Problem of Obesity." *Annual Review of Medicine.* 1981. 32:221–31.

9. Louderback L. *Fat Power, Whatever You Weigh is Right.* New York: Hawthorn Books, Inc., 1970.

10. Lewis, Susan Alice. *Perception of Body Size in 5- to 6-year-old Girls.* Salt Lake City: Thesis in Eccles Library, 1988. u.p.

11. Schwartz, MB, HO Chambliss, KD Brownell, SN Blair, C Billington. *Weight Bias Among Health Professionals Specializing in Obesity.* Ob Research Vol. 11 No. 9. Sept. 2003 1033-39.

12. Schulz, Mona Lisa. *Awakening Intuition.* New York: Random House, 1999.

13. Warner, C. Terry Ph.D. *Bonds of Anguish/Bonds of Love.* Brigham Young University, Provo, Utah. Unpublished manuscript available in the copy center. Kimball Tower, 1995.

14. McGraw, Phil. *As heard on his television show, Dr. Phil.* 2003.

15. Northrup, Christiane M.D. *Women's Bodies, Women's Wisdom,* 2nd ed. New York: Bantam Books. 1999.

16. Ibid.

CHAPTER 3

1. Dellinger, Patchen, MD. "Fat Chance." *University of Washington Columns Magazine.* March 2004.

2. Mitka, Mike. "Surgery for Obesity Demand Soars Amid Scientific, Ethical Questions." *JAMA.* April 2003.

3. Sannen I, J Himpens, G Leman. "Causes of dissatisfaction in some patients after AGB, Dept. of Surgery, Dendermonde, Belgium." *Obes Surg 2001.* Oct; 11(5): 605-8.

4. Flanagan, Latham, Jr. M.D. FACS. *Understanding the Function of the Small Gastric Pouch: Application to Post-Op Teaching and Evaluation.* Oct. 2003 Cited at www.obesitysurgery-info.com/understandings-mallgastricpouch.htm.

5. Feit H, MR Glasberg. "Neurologic complications of gastric partitioning." *Arch Neurol*, Jul 1986; 43: 642.

6. Andersen, T., OG Backer, KH Stokholm, F Quaade. "Randomized trial of diet and Gastroplasty compared with diet alone in morbid obesity." *N Engl J Med*. Feb. 9, 1984. Vol. 310:352-356.

7. Mann, Denise. "Wider Use for Obesity Surgery Urged." July 2001 *WebMd. Medical News Archives.*

8. Ravussin, Eric. "Cellular Sensors of Feast and Famine." *American Society for Clinical Investigation.* June 15, 2002. 109 (12) 1537–40.

9. Dellinger, Patchen, MD. "Fat Chance." *University of Washington Columns Magazine.* March 2004.

10. Clark, G. Wesley, M.D. *Regarding Surgical Mortality Statistics.* 2003. www.obesitysurgery-info.com/surgicalmortalitygwclark.htm.

11. Dickhaut SC, JC Delec, CP Page. "Importance of Predicting Wound Healing after Amputation." *Journal of Joint Surgery.* 1984. 66-A71-75.

12. Kay SP, Moreland JR, Schmitter E. "Nutritional Status and Wound Healing in Lower Extremity Amputations." *Clinical Orthopedics.* 1997. 217:253–56.

13. Mason, Edward E. M.D. Ph.D. "Mortality in Obesity Surgery." *Spring 2003. IBSR Newsletter.* Vol 18 No. 1. www.surgery.uiowa.edu/ ibsr.

14. Ibid.

15. Livingston, Edward. "AMA says still ethical and scientific questions with weight loss surgery." *JAMA*, April 9, 2003. Vol. 289 No. 14 pp. 1761–2.

CHAPTER 4

1. Blair, SN and RS Paffenberger. "Influence of Body Weight and Shape Variation on Incidence of Cardiovascular Disease, Diabetes, Lung Disease and Cancer." Harvard Alumni Data: Paper presented at 34th Annual Conference of Cardiovascular Disease Epidemiology and Prevention. Mar. 16–19. 1994.

2. Bailey, Covert. *The Ultimate Fit or Fat*. (New York: Houghton Mifflin, 1999).

3. Paffenberger RS, M.D. and RT Hyde, AL Wind, IM Lee, DL Jung, and JB Kamper. "The Association of Changes in Physical Activity Level and Other Lifestyle Characteristics with Mortality Among Men." *N Engl J Med* 1993. 328: 538–45.

4. Gaesser, Glenn A. Ph.D. *Big Fat Lies, The Truth about Your Weight and Your Health*. New York: Fawcett-Columbine Books, 1996.

5. Sadovsky, Richard. M.D. "Gastric Bypass Improves Diabetes and Hypertension." *Am Fam Phy*. Feb. 15, 2004.

6. Blair, SN and RS Paffenberger. "Influence of Body Weight and Shape Variation on Incidence of Cardiovascular Disease, Diabetes, Lung Disease and Cancer." Harvard Alumni Data: Paper presented at 34th Annual Conference of Cardiovascular Disease Epidemiology and Prevention. Mar. 16–19. 1994.

7. Wurtman J. *Managing Your Mind and Mood Through Food*. New York: Harper and Row, 1988.

8. Knittle, JL and K Timmeis, F Ginsberg-Feller, RE Brown and DP Katz. "The Growth of Adipose Tissue in Children and Adolescents." *Journal of Clinical Investigation*. 1979. 63:239–46.

9. Gortmaker, SL, A Must, JM Perrin, AM Sobol and WH Dietz. "Social and Economic Consequences of Overweight in Adolescence and Young Adulthood." *N Engl J Med*. 1983. 329 (14): 1008–12.

10. Dietz, WH and SL Gortmaker. "Do We Fatten Our Children at the Television Set?" *Pediatrics*. 1985. 75: 807–12.

11. Latner JD, AJ Stunkard. "Getting Worse: The Stigmatization of Obese Children." *Obesity Research*. March 2003 11(3): 452–6.

12. Lewis, Susan Alice. "Perception of Body Size in 5- to 6-Year-Old Girls." *Master's thesis, University of Utah, 1988. u.p.*

CHAPTER 5

1. Gaesser, Glenn A. Ph.D. *Big Fat Lies, The Truth About Your Weight and Your Health.* New York: Fawcett-Columbine Books, 1996.

2. Smith, Joseph. "The Word of Wisdom." *Doctrine and Covenants 1833.* Sec. 89.

3. Gaesser, Glenn A. Ph.D. and Karla Dougherty. *The Spark, The Revolutionary 3-Week Fitness Plan that Changes Everything You Know about Exercise, Weight Control and Health.* New York: Simon and Schuster, 2001.

4. Walford R.L. "The Calorically Restricted Low-Fat Nutrient-Dense Diet in Biosphere 2 Significantly Lowers Blood Glucose, Total Leukocyte Count, Cholesterol, and Blood Pressure in Humans." *Proceedings of the National Academy of Sciences.* USA. Dec. 1, 1992.

5. Shuto, Yujin. "Hypothalamic Growth Hormone Secretagogue Receptor Regulates Growth Hormone Secretion, Feeding and Adiposity." *American Society for Clinical Investigation.* June 1, 2002.

6. Gaesser, Glenn A. Ph.D. *Big Fat Lies, The Truth About Your Weight and Your Health.* New York. Fawcett-Columbine Books. 1996.

7. Peikin, Steven R. M.D. *The Complete Book of Diet Drugs.* New York: Kensington, 2000.

8. Scopinaro, Nicola M.D. *The Physiology of Weight Gain.* Italy. University of Genoa Medical School. www.obesity-online.com/ifso/lecture_Scopinaro.htm.

9. Gaesser, Glenn A. Ph.D. and Karla Dougherty. *The Spark, The Revolutionary 3-Week Fitness Plan that Changes Everything You Know about Exercise, Weight Control and Health.* New York: Simon and Schuster, 2001.

10. Ibid.

11. Flum, David, M.D. "Fat Chance." *University of Washington Columns Magazine.* March 2004.

CHAPTER 6

1. Mitchell, Deborah R, and David C Dodson. *The Diet Pill Guide.* New York: St. Martin's Griffin. 2002.

2. Ibid.

3. Peikin, Steven R. M.D. *The Complete Book of Diet Drugs.* New York: Kensington Books, 2000.

4. Mitchell, Deborah R, and David C Dodson. *The Diet Pill Guide.* New York: St. Martin's Griffin, 2002.

5. Ibid.

6. Peikin, Steven R. M.D. *The Complete Book of Diet Drugs.* New York: Kensington Books, 2000.

7. Ibid.

8. Brown, Marie-Annette, Ph.D. Jo Robinson. *When Your Body Gets the Blues.* Emmaus, Pennsylvania: Rodale Press, distributed by St. Martin's Press, 2002.

9. Haney, Daniel. "New Pill Could Attack Twin Killers." Associated Press. Mar. 10, 2004

10. United Press International. *Anti-Epilepsy Drug Fights Depression and Weight.* May 7, 2001.

11. Yang, Koseke, et. al. "Eating-related increase of dopamine concentration in the LHA with oronasal stimulation." 1996. *American Journal of Physiology* 270:R315–8.

CHAPTER 7

1. Gaesser, Glenn A. Ph.D. *Big Fat Lies, The Truth About Your Weight and Your Health.* New York: Fawcett-Columbine Books, 1996.

2. Keys, Ancel, J Brozek, A Henschel, O Michelson, HL Taylor. *Biology of Human Starvation.* Minneapolis: University of Minnesota Press, 1950.

3. Gaesser, Glenn A. Ph.D. *Big Fat Lies, The Truth About Your Weight and Your Health.* New York: Fawcett-Columbine Books, 1996.

4. Luke, HC, J Berg. *Longitudinal Birth Register Study.* 1973–95. British Medical Journal. Dec. 8, 2001.

5.   Mason, Edward E. M.D, Ph.D. "Ghrelin." *IBSR Newsletter Summer 2002.* Vol. 17. No. 2. www.surgery.uiowa.edu/ibsr.

CHAPTER 8

1.   Bouchard, C. "Is Weight Fluctuation A Risk Factor?" *N Engl J Med.* 1991. 324:1887–89.

2.   Simpson, Terry M.D. *Weight Loss Surgery Release Form.* Supplied by Kaiser Permanante. See Appendix II. obesitysurgery-info.com/wls_release_form.htm.

3.   Northrup, Christiane M.D. *Women's Bodies, Women's Wisdom,* 2nd ed. New York: Bantam Books, 1999.

4.   Bailey, Covert. *The Ultimate Fit or Fat.* New York: Houghton Mifflin, 1999.

5.   Kral, John. "Surgical Reduction of Adipose Tissue Hypercellularity in Man." *Scandinavian Journal of Plastic and Reconstructive Surgery.* 1975 9:140–43.

6.   Gaesser, Glenn A. Ph.D. *Big Fat Lies, The Truth About Your Weight and Your Health.* New York: Fawcett-Columbine Books, 1996.

7.   Malmberg, Carl. *Diet and Die.* New York: Hillman-Curl, 1935.

8.   Gaesser, Glenn A. Ph.D. *Big Fat Lies, The Truth About Your Weight and Your Health.* New York: Fawcett-Columbine Books, 1996.

9.   Rose, Laura. Life Isn't Weighed on the Bathroom Scales. Waco, Tex.: WRS Publishing, 1994.

10. Stimson, Karen, W. "Fat Feminist Herstory, 1969–1993: A Personal Memoir." *Expository Magazine.* Vol. 1, Issue 1. 2002.

CHAPTER 9

1.   Calle, Eugenia, E Michael, J Thun, Jennifer M. Petrelli, Carmen Rodriguez, and Clark W. Heath Jr. "Body Mass Index and Mortality in a Prospective Cohort of U.S. Adults." *N Engl J Med.* 1999. 341 (15): 1097–1105.

2. Stevens, J, JE Keil, PF Rust, RR Verdugo, CE Davis, HA Tyroler, and PC Gazes. "Body Mass Index and Body Girths as Predictors of Mortality in Black and White Men." *American Journal of Epidemiology.* 1992. 135: 1137–46.

3. Bailey, Covert. *The Ultimate Fit or Fat.* New York: Houghton Mifflin, 1999.

CHAPTER 10

1. Gaesser, Glenn A. Ph.D. *Big Fat Lies, The Truth About Your Weight and Your Health.* New York. Fawcett-Columbine Books. 1996.

2. Ibid.

3. Wiswell, Grant M. "Glucose Rebound following Maximal Exercise in Master Athletes." Provo, Utah Thesis in Brigham Young University Library. 2001. u.p.

4. Gaesser, Glenn A. Ph.D. and Karla Dougherty. *The Spark, The Revolutionary 3-Week fitness Plan That Changes Everything You Know About Exercise, Weight Control, and Health.* New York: Simon and Schuster, 2001.

5. Matsuzawa, Y, I Shimomura, T Nakamura, Y Keno, and K Tokunaga. *Pathophysiology and pathogenesis of visceral fat obesity.* Annual New York Academy Sciences. 1993. 676:270-78.

6. Blair, SN and RS Paffenberger. "Influence of Body Weight and Shape Variation on Incidence of Cardiovascular Disease, Diabetes, Lung Disease and Cancer." *Harvard Alumni Data: Paper presented at 34th Annual Conference of Cardiovascular Disease epidemiology and Prevention.* March 16-19, 1994 u.p.

7. Gaesser, Glenn A. Ph.D. *Big Fat Lies, The Truth About Your Weight and Your Health.* New York: Fawcett-Columbine Books, 1996.

8. Warner, C. Terry. *Bonds That Make Us Free.* Salt Lake City: The Arbinger Institute, 2001.

9. Hawks, Steven R. Ph.D. *Making Peace With the Image in the Mirror.* Salt Lake City: Bookcraft, 2001.

10. Maxwell, Neal A. *The Smallest Part.* Salt Lake City: Deseret Book, 1973.

11. Dobson, James. *What Wives Wish Their Husbands Knew About Women.* Wheaton, IL: Tyndale House Publishers, 1975.

12. Hawks, Steven R. Ph.D. *Making Peace With the Image in the Mirror.* Salt Lake City: Bookcraft, 2001.

13. Ibid.

CHAPTER 14

1. Williams, Sophia. *Minority Women and Self Esteem.* City University, Tacoma, WA. Dissertation 1995. u.p.

Index

E

DATE DUE

DEC 0 5 2007		
3/26/08 ILL		
10/27/09 ILL		